Learning Strategies for Health Careers Students

Revised Edition

Learning Strategies for Health Careers Students

Revised Edition

Susan Marcus Palau, MA
Learning Center Teacher
Cooke Center for Learning and Development
New York, NY

Marilyn Meltzer, MA
Curriculum Coordinator
Ramaz Lower School
New York, NY

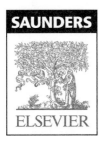

SAUNDERS

ELSEVIER

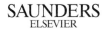

SAUNDERS
ELSEVIER

11830 Westline Industrial Drive
St. Louis, Missouri 63146

LEARNING STRATEGIES FOR HEALTH CAREERS STUDENTS
Revised Edition

ISBN-13: 978-1-4160-4270-9
ISBN-10: 1-4160-4270-9

Previous edition copyrighted 1996

ISBN-13: 978-1-4160-4270-9
ISBN-10: 1-4160-4270-9

Acquisitions Editor: Loren Wilson
Book Production Manager: Linda McKinley
Project Manager: Stephen Bancroft
Design Manager: Mark Oberkrom

Printed in the United States of America

Last digit is the print number: 9 8 7 6 5 4 3 2

To my Mother
and the memory of my Father
SMP

In memory of my Mother,
Esther Cohen Astalos
MM

Preface

Learning Strategies for Health Careers Students is intended for those health care students who need additional help in reading the textbook, writing school and work-related reports, solving math problems, and studying. The purpose of this book is to provide these students with the learning strategies that will enable them to successfully finish their health care programs and to function well in the workplace. With this book, health care students can practice basic reading, writing, math, and study skills on materials taken from currently used health care textbooks in a wide variety of fields.

Organization

Unit I, Reading Strategies, will teach students better techniques for understanding what they read. They will learn ways of organizing the vast amount of information they will be getting from their texts and ways of learning the new terminology they will be exposed to as students in health care.

Unit II, Writing Strategies, will present students with the procedures for writing reports for classroom and work purposes. Students will be shown the various processes for getting started, producing the first copy, editing for errors, and writing the final copy.

Unit III, Mathematics Strategies, will introduce students to the basic concepts of health care mathematics. These strategies should help them overcome any anxiety or resistance they may have to math.

Unit IV, Study Strategies, will provide the student with all the strategies they will need to perform well in class and on examinations.

Unit V, Reading Selections, contains 15 reading selections taken from health care textbooks and will allow the students to practice all the major strategies they learned in the other units.

Each chapter in Units I through IV contains the following:

- Learning objectives
- Vocabulary words
- Vocabulary check
- Strategies presentations
- Examples
- Exercises
- Chapter summary

Unit V, Reading Selections, gives students the chance to practice the following strategies they learned in the previous four units:

- Previewing
- Developing vocabulary
- Reading
- Writing
- Answering objective questions
- Solving word problems

Using the Textbook

Since this textbook contains 15 chapters, it is intended to be used in one semester with the students doing one chapter weekly. Unit V, Reading Selections, can be used at the same time the students are working on the chapters or when the students have finished Chapter 15.

Learning Strategies for Health Careers Students can be used in one of three ways:

1. It can be used in the traditional classroom setting with an instructor explaining and modeling the strategies to be learned.
2. Students can use this text for self-study, since the strategies are clearly explained and abundant examples are given for each strategy.
3. Students can form small groups to use this book, with an instructor acting as a consultant to these groups.

Setting Up the Course

Learning Strategies for Health Careers Students can be used by students who may have had difficulties with entrance examinations or standardized reading tests. The course can be a requirement for all incoming freshman students. This book is especially helpful for older adult students returning to school after a long time. Instructors will find this text useful for introducing all students to a higher level of academic work.

If *Learning Strategies for Health Careers Students* is used in a traditional class setting, the instructor should provide guided practice — working closely with students initially and then gradually allowing the student to work independently. If students are using this text individually or in small groups, they are encouraged to do each chapter in the given order. However, the first four units are independent of each other and can be done in any order. The instructor can be responsible for grading and assessing the students' progress or the students can assess their own progress individually or in small groups. Finally, an answer key at the end of the book will make doing this task easier.

Motivating the Students

The strategies in *Learning Strategies for Health Careers Students* are presented in a straightforward manner so that students will be successful using this book. Once they have had ample time to use these strategies in the classroom and workplace and get positive results, motivational problems for the students should be resolved.

Acknowledgments

We would like to extend a hearty thanks to Lisa Biello, Editor-in-Chief Health-Related Professions, for her good sense and great laugh. In addition, we would like to thank Margaret M. Biblis for first taking on this project. We also would like to thank Sara Meltzer and Michael Meltzer for their extraordinary word processing skills, and Mary Espenschied and Jeanne Gulledge of CRACOM Corporation who helped us in the production process.

Susan Marcus Palau
Marilyn Meltzer

Contents

Learning Strategies for Health Careers Students

Revised Edition

UNIT
I

READING STRATEGIES

As a student of the allied health professions, one of your first responsibilities will be to grapple with a great amount of reading. In many instances, this will be the first time that you will have been exposed to medical vocabulary and concepts. Because your time is so precious, it will be necessary that you get the meaning of what you are reading as efficiently as possible. You will have to recognize and understand important facts and details and apply them to real-life situations. You will have to develop a new vocabulary for your future career and learn ways of becoming aware of when you do not understand these new words and ideas from your textbook. Lastly, you will have to familiarize yourself with the layout of a textbook so that you can learn the strategies for being an active reader.

Chapter 1, Identifying the Three Levels of Understanding, will teach you how to read for a purpose. You will also be taught the strategies for reading and interpreting factual information, and for applying these new ideas to real life situations. Chapter 2, Recognizing Details, will teach you the organization of the many facts in a passage so that your comprehension will improve. Chapter 3, Developing Vocabulary, will offer you strategies for improving your medical and general vocabulary. Chapter 4, Monitoring and Improving Comprehension, will suggest ways in which you can become aware of when you are not understanding what you are reading and strategies to correct this. Finally, Chapter 5, Reading the Textbook, will explain the layout of textbooks and give you strategies for becoming an active reader of your health care texts.

Once you have completed the exercises in Unit 1, Reading Strategies, you should be better equipped to meet the first big challenge of your health care program, reading and comprehending your reading assignments as effectively as you can.

BUTTON TO MONITOR COMPREHENSION

To improve your comprehension, you must first become aware of when you are not understanding. You do this by asking yourself frequently if you are understanding what you are reading. To help you get used to monitoring your comprehension, the following button will appear throughout the text:

This button will act as a reminder to monitor your comprehension by asking yourself if you are comprehending what you are reading.

Chapter
1

Identifying the
Three Levels of
Understanding

LEARNING OBJECTIVES

In this Chapter you will learn how to
- Improve your reading comprehension by reading for a purpose
- Identify the appropriate level of understanding that fits your purpose for reading
- Use the strategies for reading at the literal, interpretive, and applied levels

VOCABULARY WORDS

The following vocabulary words are important to your understanding of the ideas in this chapter. These vocabulary words are <u>underscored</u> the first time they are used in the chapter. Read the list of words and definitions. Then check your understanding of these words before you read the chapter.

asepsis the absence of germs (Mosby's Dictionary, p. 150).

autocratic pertaining to one who has total power.

conclusions outcomes or results.

document informational paper.

efficiently pertaining to being productive without any waste.

hemostasis stopping blood flow by natural and artificial means.

lymph a thin watery fluid originating in the organs and tissues of the body that circulates through the lymphatic vessels and is filtered by the lymph nodes (Mosby's Dictionary, p. 1123).

neurologist a physician who specializes in the nervous system and its disorders (Mosby's Dictionary, p. 1283).

supine lying horizontally on the back (Mosby's Dictionary, p. 1795).

topical pertaining to the surface of a part of the body (Mosby's Dictionary, p. 1866).

VOCABULARY CHECK

Directions: Choose the vocabulary word that best fits into the sentence.

1. The unit coordinator prided himself on working as _EFFICIENTLY_ as possible.

2. In the operating room, the principles of _ASEPSIS_ are applied.

3. One of the major fluids in the human body is the _LYMPH_.

4. The pharmacist sold me over-the-counter _TOPICAL_ medicine to put on my sunburn.

5. I saw a _NEUROLOGIST_ after I had a severe headache for over a month.

6. Before surgery, the orderly placed the patient on the operating table in the _SUPINE_ position.

7. Her _AUTOCRATIC_ personality in the classroom made her young students dislike her.

8. In order to manage the patient during the operation, the technician maintained _HEMOSTATIS_.

9. He typed a copy of the _DOCUMENT_ on the computer.

10. The two mystery stories with the same name ended with different _CONCLUSIONS_

READING WITH A PURPOSE

As students in the health care professions, you quickly discover the great amount of reading that you are required to complete. It is necessary that you accomplish these reading tasks as <u>efficiently</u> as possible. This means that you get as much understanding as you can during each of your study sessions. You cannot afford to waste time by performing at less than your best each time you sit at your desk and read. An excellent strategy that guarantees that each reading session will be successful is to read with a purpose. When you read with a purpose, you create a goal that you wish to accomplish each time you read. Having a goal to reach will keep you focused and involved in your reading. Your comprehension will be improved by reading with a purpose.

INTRODUCING THE THREE LEVELS OF UNDERSTANDING

There is more than one way to understand what you are reading in your textbook. The goal or purpose you set for yourself as you read will determine the level of understanding required for comprehension of the reading material.

- The first level of understanding is called **literal understanding**. This level of understanding requires that you know what the subject of your reading is and the most important points being made about the subject. For example, when you need to learn important terms, names and functions of different parts of the body, or steps in a procedure from your textbook, you use literal understanding.
- The second level of understanding is called **interpretive understanding**. This level of understanding requires that you draw <u>conclusions</u> about what you are reading by examining the facts that are presented. For example, when you are reading to learn how to schedule patients according to the seriousness of their complaints, reading to learn how to decide on the proper medical insurance forms to fill out for a patient, or reading to learn how to examine stained smears for the presence of certain microorganisms, you use interpretive understanding.
- The third level of understanding is called **applied understanding**. This level of understanding requires that you see how ideas are similar so that you can use ideas from one situation in another related situation. For example, when you are asked to read a chapter about focusing the microscope and then you use one correctly in the laboratory or when you memorize from your text the proper hand-washing technique and then use it when you handle patients, you use applied understanding.

Again, your goal or purpose for reading will determine which level of understanding you need to use when reading your textbook.

EXERCISE 1–1

Directions: Your instructor gives you assignments to learn different types of information. These assignments are listed below. If the assignment requires literal understanding, write "L" in the blank next to the assignment. If the assignment requires interpretive understanding, write "I" in the blank next to the assignment. If the assignment requires applied understanding, write "A" in the blank next to the assignment.

Assignment 1: You are asked to memorize the names of the important parts of the human brain. _L_

Assignment 2: You are asked to make up a patient chart following a model chart that the instructor has created. _A_

Assignment 3: The instructor asks you to retype a document that has been corrected and marked with proofreading symbols. I

Assignment 4: You are asked to figure out what the different tail positions of a cat mean. I

Assignment 5: You are given a chart of the components of blood and are asked to label the different parts. L

Assignment 6: The instructor hands you a study sheet describing the different plural endings of medical terms. You are asked to use the plural endings for every medical term in a report you are writing. A

Assignment 7: After successfully completing Chapter 9 in your textbook, you are expected to be able to fill a syringe. A

Assignment 8: You are expected to spell all the important words in the first chapter of your health care textbook. L

Assignment 9: You are asked to list the six sections of the Food Guide Pyramid. L

Assignment 10: You need to determine whether a patient's diet includes all sections of the Food Guide Pyramid. I

Let us now take a closer look at each of the different levels of understanding and see how each level suggests a strategy for improving reading comprehension.

Literal Understanding

When you read for literal understanding, you are reading for facts and information. You are trying to determine what the passage is saying in a basic, straightforward way. The strategy to use for literal understanding is to identify the topic and main idea of the selection you are reading. Finding the topic and main idea of a passage will give you a purpose for reading and will help you to concentrate on the essential points in the selection that you need to learn.

Identifying the Topic of a Passage

The topic is the key subject of the passage. To find the topic, you ask:

- What is this passage mostly about?

The answer will be the topic or subject of the passage and should be stated as briefly as possible.

Example 1–1

Following is a selection from Solomon (p. 199). Read the passage and notice how one reader identified the topic of the passage by asking, What is this passage mostly about?

By filtering and destroying bacteria from the lymph, the lymph nodes help prevent the spread of infection. When bacteria are present, lymph nodes may increase in size and become tender. For example, you may have experienced the swollen cervical lymph nodes that often accompany a sore throat. An infection in almost any part of the body may result in swelling and tenderness of the lymph nodes that drain that area.

- Question: What is this passage mostly about?
- Answer: lymph nodes = Topic.

Notice also that the term *lymph nodes* appears many times in the selection. A repeated word is also a clue that the topic of the passage is "lymph nodes."

EXERCISE 1-2

Directions: Read the following selections. In the space provided, write the topic of each selection. Remember to use the strategy of asking yourself, What is this passage mostly about? Be as brief as possible with your answer. Check to see if the word or words you choose appear frequently in the selection.

1. The health unit coordinator has access to a great deal of *protected health information (PHI)* because of the very nature of the job. Protected health information is information about the patient that includes demographic information (e.g., name, address, phone number) that may identify the individual and relates to his or her past, present, or future physical or mental health and related health care services. This information must be treated with absolute confidentiality by all health personnel (LaFleur Brooks and Gillingham, p. 83).

Topic: PROTECTED HEALTH INFORMATION (PHI)

2. Hemostasis is a physiologic response to arrest bleeding. Various surgical techniques can be used to augment this physiologic clotting process. The surgical assistant should be able to perform or to assist with routine hemostatic procedures.

   Excellent hemostasis is vital (1) to obtain optimal visibility at the surgical site, (2) to limit the volume of blood loss, and (3) to decrease risk of infection (extravasated blood is an ideal medium for bacterial growth) (McCurnin, p. 724).

Topic: HEMOSTASIS

3. It is always advisable to carefully check all references and to follow through on any leads for information. It is best to use the telephone in checking references, because people are sometimes less than candid in a letter; furthermore, letter writing is time consuming and a reply may never be sent (Young and Kennedy, p. 387).

Topic: CHECKING REFERENCES BY PHONE

4. Use of the cat has increased in psychotherapy sessions to stimulate communication, provide an object for affection, and allow the patient's mastery of a situation. Cats have also been prescribed for home therapy, working 24 hours a day to draw individuals into an awareness of their surroundings or provide affection and emotional security where it might be lacking. Therapy in institutional settings for the emotionally disturbed and mentally retarded has also received a big boost when cats are part of the settings, because the animals increase the effect of the professional staff and provide continuity during staff turnovers (Beaver, p. 7-8).

Topic: USE OF A CAT; PSYCHOTHERAPY

5. Appointment scheduling is the process that determines which patients will be seen by the physician, the dates and times of appointments, and how much time will be allotted to each patient based on his or her complaint, as well as the physician's availability. Time management involves the realization that there will always be unforeseen interruptions and delays. Most providers of medical care find that efficient scheduling of appointments is one of the most important factors in the success of the practice. There are many approaches to scheduling, and each facility must find what suits it best (Young and Kennedy, p. 166).

Topic: APPOINTMENTS

Identifying the Main Idea

The main idea of a passage is what the passage is all about. The strategy to use to identify the main idea is to ask,

- What is the most important point being made about the topic?

The answer will be the main idea and should be stated in sentence form.

Example 1–2

Read the following excerpt from a health care textbook and pay attention to how the reader found the main idea by identifying the topic and then asking the question, What is the most important point being made about the topic?

Good business writing depends on clarity. If the basic element used to convey meaning—the sentence—is unclear, the entire message may be difficult to understand. Good sentence structure requires the application of all the rules of English grammar and the avoidance of certain particularly common errors. (Diehl, p. 356).

- What is this passage mostly about? Good writing = Topic.
- What is the most important point being made about good writing? Good writing depends on clear sentences = Main idea.

Notice that the first sentence in the paragraph, "Good business writing depends on clarity," contains the main idea of the selection. In this example the main idea was the first sentence. In other cases, however, the main idea may be in the last sentence, in the middle sentence, or in both the first and last sentences. In some instances, you may not be able to find a main idea sentence. In such cases, you will need to create your own main idea sentence. The strategy will be the same as you used for finding a given main idea sentence. You determine the topic and then ask the main idea question: What is the most important point being made about the topic? As long as you use this strategy, your answer should lead you to the main idea, regardless of where it is located. As long as you create and answer the main idea question, you should be able to make up your own main idea if one cannot be found in the passage.

EXERCISE 1–3

Directions: Read the following passages taken from health care textbooks. In the space provided, write in the topic and underline the main idea sentence. If the main idea is not stated, create your own in the space provided. In either case, don't forget to use the strategy of asking yourself the two questions:

- What is this passage mostly about? = Topic
- What is the most important point being made about the topic = Main idea

Don't forget that the main idea sentence can appear anywhere in the passage, or not at all.

1. The cell is the basic unit of all living things. The human body is made up of trillions of cells. Cells perform specific functions, and their size and shape vary according to function. Bones, muscles, skin, and blood are each made up of different kinds of cells. Body cells are

microscopic; approximately 2,000 are needed to make an inch (LaFleur Brooks and Gillingham, p. 447).

Topic: _CELLS_

(Unstated main idea: _WHAT CELLS ARE_)

2. Three types of connective tissue fibers are collagen fibers, reticular fibers, and elastic fibers. **Collagen fibers** are the most numerous. These fibers contain the protein collagen, the most abundant protein in the body. Collagen is a very tough substance, and **collagen** fibers give great strength to body structures. (Solomon, p. 33).

Topic: _FIBERS_

(Unstated main idea: _DEF. OF COLLAGEN FIBERS_

3. Topical anesthetics, which are formulated as a highly concentrated gel, provide a temporary numbing effect on the nerve endings on the surface of the oral mucosa. Only small amounts of topical anesthetic should be applied to the limited area being treated (Robinson and Bird, p. 193).

Topic: _TOPICAL ANESTHETICS_

(Unstated main idea: _USAGE OF TOPICAL ANESTHETICS_

4. Inside the casing of the main computer hardware, the microprocessor is housed. The microprocessor is the central unit of the computer that contains the logic circuitry, which carries out the instructions of a computer's programs. It is considered the most important piece of hardware in a computer system. Microprocessors act as the brain of the computer and interpret instructions from a program (Young and Kennedy, p. 135).

Topic: _MICROPROCESSOR_

(Unstated main idea: _FUNCTION OF MICROPROCESSOR_

5. The surgical site is usually prepared after the animal is anesthetized. The hair is first clipped in the same direction as the hair growth. Then it is clipped against the direction of growth to achieve the closest shave possible (using a no. 40 clipper blade). A wide region of skin is clipped around the proposed surgical incision. A general rule is to shave at least 2 to 4 cm in every direction from the proposed incision, depending on the size of the animal and location of the incision. For abdomninal procedures, the clip should extend several centimeters cranial to the xyphoid, caudal to the pubis, and lateral to the nipples. For orthopedic procedures, the entire circumference of the limb is clipped from the foot up onto the body. Long hair growing near the periphery of the clipped area should be cut short enough that it cannot hang over the clipped area. Sterile, water-soluble lubricant may be placed in open wounds before clipping around them. The lubricant will collect hair, allowing it to be rinsed away before the surgical scrub. Areas that appear to be infected should be clipped last so the clippers do not spread infected material. After clipping, a vacuum cleaner may be used to eliminate loose hairs on the skin. The surgical clip should be thorough but gentle. Unnecessary roughness will result in inflamed or traumatized skin, which can cause greater postoperative complications.

Initial skin preparation is done in the preparation room to remove gross contamination. Before scrubbing the abdomen of a male dog, the prepuce should be flushed with an antiseptic solution. Examination gloves are worn to decrease contamination from the hands. The surgical scrub is performed by alternating an antiseptic scrub (such as povidone-iodine or chlorhexidine scrub) with alcohol or sterile saline. (Remember not to use alcohols or detergents in open wounds, eyes, or mucous membranes). Scrubbing should begin over the proposed incision site and extend outward in a spiraling pattern, never going back toward the center with the same gauze sponge. The sponge is replaced with a clean one and the process is repeated until no dirt is visible on the discarded sponges.

The sterile-surgical scrub is done once the animal is properly positioned on the operating table. Sterile gloves should be worn and sterile sponges are used. If the sterile surgical scrub is performed by alternating povidone-iodine with alcohol, the total contact time of the povidone-iodine should be at least 5 minutes. After the final povidone-iodine scrub, a 10% povidone-iodine solution should be sprayed or painted on the skin. Alternatively, the sterile surgical scrub may be performed by alternating chlorhexidine gluconate with either alcohol or sterile saline. Either chlorhexidine or sterile saline may be left on the skin at the end of preparation. Both povidone-iodine and chlorhexidine are effective scrub solutions, but the contact time for chlorhexidine is less critical than for povidone-iodine (McCurnin, p. 704).

Topic: _SURGICAL SITE ON ANIMAL_

(Unstated main idea: _PROCEDURE_)

Interpretive Understanding

When you read for interpretive understanding, you are reading to figure out something unstated in the passage. The strategy you use for interpretive understanding is to examine the facts or details in the passage and to use your own experience and background knowledge to draw a conclusion about the meaning of the passage. Drawing the correct conclusions about what you are reading will allow you to understand better what the writer really means and will allow you to function better in your workplace.

Details as Clues

When you use interpretive understanding, you need to go beyond the literal meaning of the passage and reason out in what direction the facts or details are leading. This requires that you infer or make a judgment about the meaning of the details. In other words, your responsibility when using interpretive understanding is to examine the details and use them as clues to help you form your own logical conclusions. In addition, you need to rely on information you have learned from your other classes and from your own life in order to come to the right explanation of the passage.

Example 1–3

Read the following description of a medical assistant's boss adapted from Young and Kennedy (p. 380). Then read how the medical assistant interpreted this behavior and drew the conclusion on the best way to behave with this boss. Notice that she uses facts describing the boss and her own experience to interpret the situation.

The autocratic manager is more of a dictator who leads by making demands and insisting tasks be done in a certain way—his or her way.

MEDICAL ASSISTANT'S INTERPRETIVE UNDERSTANDING:

I see that the boss is a leader. That means that he must need followers. I guess that means that I must carefully follow whatever orders he gives me. I see that he likes to tell you how and when to do things. My dad is like that and, boy, does he get angry when I take that responsibility on myself. I'd better wait and let the boss show me how to do things around here and let him decide on my schedule. I also understand that he likes to do everything himself. I remember reading about that type of personality in my psych class.

It will be in my best interest not to seem too bossy. It seems that, to get along with this guy, I must follow all his directions and stick to the rules of the office.

Note that the medical assistant used both the details or facts describing the boss and her own personal knowledge and experience to determine what type of behavior would be best with the autocratic type of boss.

EXERCISE 1–4

Directions: Below are a series of situations taken from health care textbooks. Following each is an interpretive understanding question. Read the question and choose the best answer by circling the letter of the best choice. Remember to use facts from the passages and your own personal experience and knowledge to help you choose the correct answer.

1. Remember that the interview is centered on the medical assistant, so freely discuss the skills and attributes that will be brought to the job. Be prepared to answer questions such as "Tell me about yourself" and "Why do you want to work for this company?" (Adapted from Young and Kennedy, pp. 1236-1237).

You can conclude that the reason the interviewer starts the interview in this way is to
   a. see if you are made nervous easily
   b. have a chance to get acquainted
   c. check how well you memorized your résumé
   d. determine whether you think and talk like the interviewer

2. The physician obtains information for the history by questioning the patient or the family or persons accompanying the patient when the patient is unable to provide the history. A carefully taken history will direct the focus of the physical exam and assist with making the final diagnosis (Diehl, p. 297).

You can conclude from this that
   a. A patient with headaches will have a neurologist pay more attention to his head than his other body systems to some extent.
   b. The neurologist would not be interested in the fact that the patient hit his head 2 months ago.
   c. The neurologist would ask for a medical history only after she has examined the patient thoroughly.
   d. A general practitioner would make an automatic referral to a neurologist for this patient before examining him.

3. The treatments are performed at the patient's bedside by a respiratory therapist. It is important that the health unit coordinator enter all of the information regarding the order into the computer or onto the requisition form. The respiratory therapist will then bring the needed equipment and medication to the unit and will not have to delay the patient's treatment by having to return to obtain necessary items. The therapist will usually read the doctor's order before administering the treatment. Upon completion of the treatment, the therapist records the type of medication and treatment and other pertinent data on a respiratory therapy record sheet on the patient's chart.

To communicate the doctor's order to the respiratory care department, use the computer or complete a respiratory care requisition (LaFleur Brooks and Gillingham, p. 338).

Which of the following questions does the passage answer?
a. Who is responsible for writing in the patient's chart?
b. What respiratory treatments are the best?
c. What medications did the doctor order?
d. Who is responsible for communicating with the respiratory department?

4. Routine samples are collected in clean, dry containers, but urine needed for bacterial culture is collected in sterile containers. Samples that cannot be analyzed within 30 minutes of collection should be refrigerated in airtight containers. Once they have been refridgerated, urine specimens should be returned to room temperature before urinalysis is performed (McCurnin, p. 96).

You can conclude that
a. The proper collection and handling of urine for culture is important.
b. You should collect urine only by catheterization.
c. Because there is bacteria in urine, it does not need refrigeration.
d. All of the above.

5. For vision to occur, light must pass through the eye and form an image on the retina. Light must pass through several layers of connecting neurons in the retina to reach the rods and cones (Solomon, p. 131).

Which of the following statements can be concluded from the passage?
a. The only organ involved with seeing is the eye.
b. The retina does not have nerve endings.
c. Light is crucial to seeing.
d. The retina is the first part of the eye that light reaches.

EXERCISE 1–5

Read the following excerpt on minimizing waiting time for a patient on the telephone (Young and Kennedy, p. 150). Using your background knowledge and experience and details from the passage, write the best responses in the spaces provided.

When a call cannot be put through immediately, ask,

Will you wait, or should I have the Dr. call you back?

If the caller elects to wait, remember that waiting with a silent telephone can be irritating and **tedious**. The waiting time always seems long, no matter how brief it really is. Many of today's phones are equipped with timers that tell the caller exactly how long they have been waiting on hold. The longer they wait, the more irritated they may become. Let no more than 1 minute pass without breaking in with some reassuring comment. For instance,

I'm sorry, but the Dr. is still busy.

If the wait is longer than expected, the caller may wish to reconsider and call back at another time or have the call returned. By going back on the line at frequent intervals, the caller has an opportunity to express such concerns. Ask the caller if he or she wishes to continue waiting. The medical assistant could say,

I'm sorry that you are waiting so long. Would you like me to return your call when the Dr. is free?

Try to give the caller some estimate of when he or she may expect the return call. In any event, be considerate and remember that irritation can be lessened each time the medical assistant returns to the call by saying,

Thank you for waiting.

When it is necessary to leave the telephone and obtain information, ask the caller:

Will you please wait while I get the information?

Listen for a reply. If it will take longer than a few seconds to get the information, give some estimate of the time required and offer to call back. When returning to the telephone, always thank the caller for waiting.

Applied Understanding

When you read for applied understanding, you are reading to learn ideas from your textbook so you can use these ideas in school or in the workplace. The strategies you will use for applied understanding include the strategies you use for literal and interpretive understanding.

- In order to apply information, you must first learn the facts. This will require that you learn and remember ideas literally. Finding the topic and the main idea will help you focus on what is important.
- In order to apply information, you must be able to interpret what you are reading. This will require that you have some background knowledge of the subject and of the situation to which you will be applying the information.
- Finally, in order to apply information, you must use good judgment. You must be able to recognize the similarities and differences between the facts you read and the situations in which you will be applying these facts. You must be able to judge when and where it is appropriate and correct to apply these facts. This judgment requires that you know your facts and have experience. Following is an example adapted from Bird and Robinson (p. 478) of how one dental assistant student thought through an emergency situation and successfully used applied understanding in the workplace.

Example 1–4

Today was my third day of clinical placement and I was working with Dr. Pepper and his patients. The night before, I had finished reading Chapter 9 in my textbook, and one part of the chapter stuck in my mind—the procedure for responding to the patient who feels faint. I remember it said the following:

1. _Place the patient in a subsupine position with the head lower than the feet._
   Purpose: This position causes blood to flow away from the stomach and back toward the brain; this is frequently sufficient to revive the patient.
2. _Call for emergency assistance (911)._
3. _Loosen any binding clothes on the patient._
4. _Have an ammonia inhalant ready to administer by waving it under the patient's nose several times._
5. _Have oxygen ready to administer._
6. _Monitor and record patient's vital signs._

Was I glad that I learned this because Mrs. Klein, who must be about 6 months pregnant, appeared to faint as I raised the back of her chair. My first responsibility was to judge whether or not she had actually fainted. I called her name and she responded that she felt faint. At that point I buzzed for Dr. Pepper, while I slowly lowered the back of the chair and located the ammonia inhalant. Just as I had taken her vital signs to record and give to Dr. Pepper, he had arrived and started to give Mrs. Klein some oxygen. Dr. Pepper praised me for acting so calmly and using good judgment in an emergency situation. I was glad I knew my facts also so I was able to do the right thing.

EXERCISE 1–6

Directions: In the left-hand column are titles of chapters from a textbook by Young and Kennedy. In the right-hand column are tasks taken from Young and Kennedy that you should be able to complete after reading and learning the correct chapter. In the blank space next to the task, write in the letter of the chapter you would need to learn in order to perform the task. The first one has been done for you.

A. Infection Control (Ch. 24)

B. Banking Services and Procedures (Ch. 19)

C. Patient Reception and Processing (Ch. 11)

D. Written Communications and Mail Processing (Ch. 12)

E. Basics of Procedural Coding (Ch. 16)

F. Medical Practice Management (Ch. 20)

G. Vital Signs (Ch. 28)

H. Assisting in Ophthalmology and Otolaryngology (Ch. 34)

I. Nutrition and Health Promotion (Ch. 27)

J. Surgical Asepsis and Assisting with Surgical Procedures (Ch. 54)

K. Assisting with Medical Emergencies (Ch. 33)

___I___ Explain the difference between "good" and "bad" cholesterol (p. 498)

___G___ Obtain a patient's height and weight within 1/4 inch and 1/4 pound of your evaluator's measurements (pp. 541-544)

___D___ Address envelopes using the guidelines for optical scanning (pp. 214-216)

___A___ Perform a 2-minute medical handwash according to medical aseptic principles without missing a step or incorrectly performing a step (pp. 459-461)

___C___ List at least 10 items that should be completed on a patient's registration form (pp. 192-193)

___E___ List the steps to assign a CPT code (pp. 298-299)

___H___ Collect a throat culture and prepare it for immediate examination (p. 680)

___B___ Discuss the advantage of using checks for the transfer of funds (p. 353)

___F___ Arrange a group meeting (p. 395)

___K___ Recognize the major symptoms of a heart attack (p. 641)

___J___ Put on a pair of sterile gloves without contaminating them (pp. 1181-1184)

REVIEWING THE LEARNING STRATEGIES

TO LEARN	USE THIS STRATEGY
Literal understanding	Identify the topic of the passage by asking What is this passage mostly about?
	Identify the main idea of the passage by asking, What is the most important point being made about the topic?
Interpretive understanding	Examine the facts and details.
	Use your own experiences and background knowledge to draw conclusions.
Applied understanding	Learn the facts for literal understanding.
	Use experience and background knowledge to interpret situations.
	Use your best judgment to determine when it is appropriate to apply facts to a new situation.

Chapter
2

Recognizing Details

LEARNING OBJECTIVES

In this chapter you learn how to
- Locate details
- Distinguish between the main idea and important details
- Verify facts from the text
- Recognize logical relationships

VOCABULARY WORDS

The following vocabulary words are important to your understanding of the ideas in this chapter. These vocabulary words are underscored the first time they are used in the chapter. Read the list of words and definitions. Then check your understanding of these words before you read the chapter.

accredited credentialed.

aneurysm a sac formed by the localized dilation of the wall of an artery.

aneurysmectomy surgical removal of an aneurysm.

apprenticeship the practical experience of training under skilled workers.

beneficence kindness.

disclosure something made known.

pancreas a large gland located behind the stomach.

quadrant one of four parts.

sodium salt.

veracity truthfulness.

VOCABULARY CHECK

Directions: Choose the vocabulary word that best fits into the sentence.

1. He learned his trade as a carpenter by serving an _APPRENTICESHIP_.
2. Her _BENEFICENCE_ toward others made everyone love her.
3. Is the school that you are attending an _ACCREDITED_ institution?
4. Although hearing the truth was difficult, I appreciate the doctor's _VERACITY_.
5. The _DISCLOSURE_ of health records is unethical without the patients permission.
6. You should be on a low _SODIUM_ diet.
7. Will you measure one of the _QUADRANT_(s) of the circle?
8. The _ANEURYSM_ in his aorta was fatal.
9. The _ANEURYSMECTOMY_ is the surgery that saved his life.
10. The _PANCREAS_ is an organ of the digestive system.

LOCATING SUPPORTING DETAILS

When you are learning information in the health care fields, it is essential that you learn to locate the important details that explain, illustrate, or prove the main idea. These important details are the facts that help you to understand the main point of the reading material. These facts explain how things work, how things are made, what they are, and why things happen. Locating the supporting details and understanding how these details relate to the main idea is key to your understanding your textbooks.

DISTINGUISHING BETWEEN MAIN IDEA AND SUPPORTING DETAILS

As you read your textbooks, you concentrate on identifying the main idea. In the health care fields, understanding the important details and following the way these details develop the main idea are necessary tools to help you learn the information in your textbooks. As you read your assignments, it is important for you to be able to distinguish the main idea from the important details. Remember that the main idea is a general statement and that the details are specific facts.

MAPPING DETAILS

Details are facts and examples that give you a better understanding of the most important point of a paragraph. Details, then, will relate to or support the main idea.

There are two kinds of details—**important details** and **less important details.** **Important details** relate directly to the main idea. They describe and tell you more about the important point of a paragraph. The relationship between important details and the main idea would look like this diagram or map:

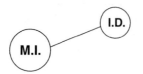

Most paragraphs from your health care textbooks will be filled with many important details. A mapping of the details would look more like this:

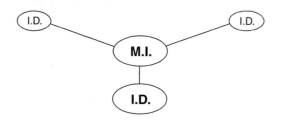

Less important details are details that relate directly to important details. They describe and tell you more about these important details. The relationship among less important details, important details, and the main idea would look like this map:

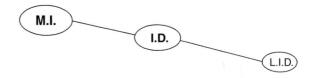

Again, paragraphs from your health care textbooks will be more complex than this. A mapping of both types of details would look more like this:

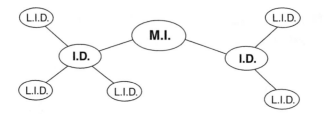

Mapping the main ideas and details will help you visualize, or see, the relationship of the important and less important details to the main idea. This will enable you to better understand what you are reading. It makes sense, especially when you are having trouble understanding a paragraph, to try this strategy. Sometimes seeing how the details relate to each other and the main idea will make the reading clear.

Example 2–1

Below is a selection from *the Young* and Kennedy health care textbook *Kinn's The Medical Assistant an Applied Learning Approach,* (p. 417). Following the passage is an example of how to map the main ideas, important details, and less important details.

As technology advanced and more health records became computerized, legislation dealing with privacy became imperative. HIPAA of 1996 was developed, in part, to help ensure the confidentiality of medical records. The statute, which became law in August of 1996, applies to those records that are created or maintained by healthcare providers, health plans, and healthcare clearinghouses that engage in certain electronic transactions.

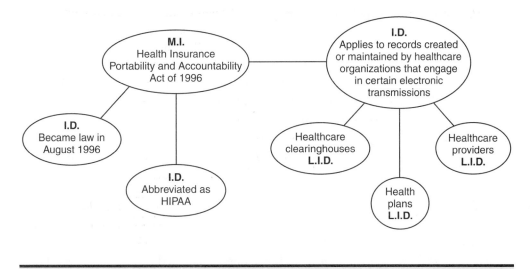

EXERCISE 2–1

Directions: Read the following selection from the Robinson and Bird health care textbook *Essentials of Dental Assisting,* (p. 83). In the space provided at the top of page 20, draw a details map showing the relationship of the main idea to the important details and less important details.

Healthy skin is better able to withstand the damaging effects of repeated washing and of wearing gloves. It is important to dry hands well before donning gloves.

Keep nails short and clean. Long nails or artificial nails are likely to harbor pathogens, puncture examination gloves, or accidentally poke a patient. In addition, microorganisms thrive around rough cuticles and can enter the body through any break in the skin.

Dental personnel with open sores or weeping dermatitis must avoid activities involving direct patient contact and handling contaminated instruments or equipment until the condition is resolved.

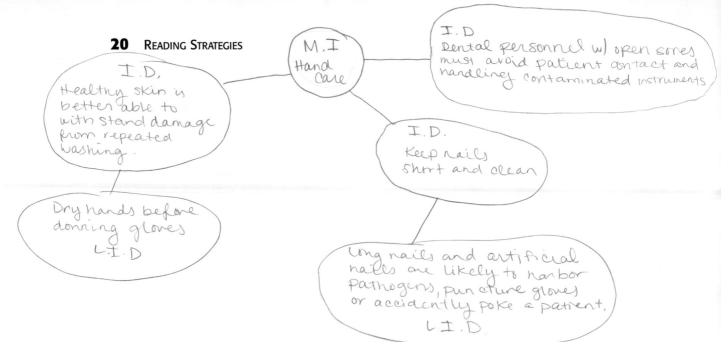

I.D
Dental personnel w/ open sores must avoid patient contact and handling contaminated instruments

M.I
Hand Care

I.D,
Healthy skin is better able to with stand damage from repeated washing.

I.D.
Keep nails short and clean

Dry hands before donning gloves
L.I.D

Long nails and artificial nails are likely to harbor pathogens, puncture gloves or accidently poke a patient.
L.I.D

VERIFYING FACTS FROM THE TEXT

When reading your textbooks, your purpose is to learn the information in the assigned chapters. You will most likely have to answer questions following the reading. These questions may be at the end of the chapter or on a study guide provided by the instructor. When you are answering these questions, you want to be able to verify, or prove, that your answers are correct by scanning back to the pages you have read in the text. Scanning for facts is an essential reading strategy that will help you use your textbook more efficiently. Focus on key words in the question to help you find the information you need in the text.

Example 2–2

Directions: Read the following excerpt adapted from a health care textbook (Bird and Robinson, p. 24). Answer the multiple-choice questions based on the selection. Then read the explanation of the answers.

THE DENTAL LABORATORY TECHNICIAN

The *dental laboratory technician* usually does not work in the dental office with the other team members, although some dental offices have "in-house" laboratories. Many dental technicians choose to be employed in private laboratories, and others choose to own and operate their own laboratory. In either case, the dental laboratory technician may legally perform only those tasks specified by the *written prescription* of the dentist.

In most states, dental laboratory technicians are not required to have formal education. They can receive their training through apprenticeship, commercial schools, or ADA-accredited programs. Many have received their training in ADA-accredited programs that are two years in length. Dental laboratory technicians have extensive knowledge of dental anatomy and materials and also excellent manual dexterity.

1. The dental laboratory technician may legally perform
   a. all the mechanical tasks of the dentist.
   b. the written information prescribed by the dental laboratory.
   c. the mechanical tasks specified by the written prescription of the dentist.
   d. none of the technical skilled tasks required by the dentist.

2. Dental laboratory technicians are employed by
   a. dental offices with "in house" laboratories.
   b. self-employed.
   c. large laboratories.
   d. all of the above.

3. Many dental laboratory technicians are in ADA-accredited training programs which are
   a. one year.
   b. two years.
   c. three years.
   d. four years.

The answer to question 1 is c. The key word in the question — *legally* — helps you to scan back to the first sentence of the passage. Read this sentence carefully, and you will be able to prove that you have chosen the correct answers. The word *all* in choice a makes that answer incorrect. Choice b is incorrect because a careful reading reveals that the information is prescribed by the *dentist*, not by the dental laboratory. Choice d is incorrect because the word *none* is too exclusive.

The answer to question 2 is d. *Employed* is the key word in the question. Use the key word to scan paragraph 2. All of the choices are correct; therefore choice d is the answer.

The answer to question 3 is b. The key word in question 3 is *training*. Scan the selection to find information about training in the third paragraph. A careful reading of the details will reveal that the information in answer choices a, c, and d are factually incorrect based on the information in the text.

EXERCISE 2–2

Directions: Read the following excerpt from a health care textbook (Bird and Robinson, pp. 37-38). Answer the multiple-choice questions based on the selection. Use key words in the question to scan back to the passage to locate the correct answer. On the line next to the question, fill in the paragraph and line number of your answer choice.

THE DUTY OF CARE

The duty of care owed by a dentist to a patient includes (1) being licensed; (2) using reasonable skill, care, and judgment; and (3) using standard drugs, materials, and techniques. The dentist may refuse to treat a patient; however, this action must *not* be based on the patient's race, color, or creed.

In addition, the Americans with Disabilities Act protects patients with infectious diseases such as human immunodeficiency virus (HIV) infection. For example, a patient with HIV cannot be refused treatment simply because of the disease. The only exception would be the HIV patient who has a special condition (e.g., severe periodontal disease) that requires the care of a specialist, and the dentist would refer any patient with the same condition to a specialist, regardless of HIV status. In other words, a patient cannot be refused treatment based *only* on HIV status.

Abandonment

Abandonment refers to discontinuation of care after treatment has begun, but before it has been completed. The dentist may be liable for abandonment if the dentist ends the dentist-patient relationship without giving the patient reasonable notice. Even if a patient refuses to follow instructions and fails to keep appointments, the dentist may not legally refuse to give the patient another appointment. The dentist may not dismiss or refuse to treat a patient of record without giving the patient written notification of termination. After notification, care must continue for a reasonable length of time, usually 30 days, to allow the patient time to find another dentist. It could even be considered abandonment if a dentist left the area for a week-end without making arrangements with another dentist to be available for emergencies, or without leaving a number for the patient to call for care.

Patient Responsibilities

The patient also has legal duties to the dentist. The patient is legally required to pay a reason-able and agreed-on fee for services. The patient also is expected to cooperate and follow instruc-tions regarding treatment and home care.

1. The duty of care owed by a dentist to a patient includes all but:
   a. being licensed.
   b. using reasonable care.
   c. giving his/her home telephone number.
   d. using standard techniques.

   par# ___1___
   line# ___2-4___

2. The patient is required to pay the dentist's fee, when the fee is
   a. set by the dentist's overhead.
   b. based on insurance payments.
   c. what the patient can afford to pay.
   d. agreed upon by the patient and the dentist.

   par# ___4___
   line# ___2-3___

3. The dentist can dismiss a patient
   a. any time.
   b. after 2 years.
   c. after giving written notice.
   d. after finding another dentist to continue the patient's treatment.

   par# ___2___
   line# ___8-10___

4. If a dentist refuses treatment, the dentist
   a. must find another dentist to treat the patient.
   b. should direct the patient to a dental clinic.
   c. must continue care for a reasonable length of time.
   d. should indicate to the patient where treatment might be received.

   par# ___2___
   line# ___5-9___

5. The drugs that a dentist uses on his patient must be
   a. standard.
   b. prescription
   c. over-the-counter.
   d. nonaddictive

   par# ___1___
   line# ___3-4___

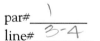

RECOGNIZING LOGICAL RELATIONSHIPS

When reading health care textbooks, you must pay close attention to details. As you read, you should think about these facts and how they are organized. Details in your textbook are grouped so that you can easily identify the relationship between the idea and details. These organizational patterns make it easier for you to remember information.

TYPES OF PATTERNS

There are patterns of organization that are often found in textbooks. Both single paragraphs and longer selections are structured in these patterns and in combinations of these patterns. When you learn to recognize these organizational patterns, you will be able to closely follow the ideas in your texts.

FOLLOWING THE ORDER OF DETAILS

When you are reading, it is important to follow the order of details. Following the order of details is important when you are studying for exams or following written directions on the job.

Correctly following the order, or steps, is necessary if you are to do your work correctly. If you confuse the order of the directions, you could make a serious mistake. To avoid these errors, pay attention to the order of details. Your first step in reading is to identify the topic and the main idea of the reading material. Details in a reading passage are put together so that readers can better understand the main idea. All the details relate to the main idea and help the reader understand the main idea.

There are words that signal you to be aware of the correct order of details. Some of these directional words are

• First	• When	• Next
• Second	• In conclusion	• After
• Last	• Then	• During
• Finally	• Before	• Following

Just as traffic signals help you to follow the correct road when you travel, directional words help you to stay on track and follow the correct order of the details. Paying attention to the order of details helps you to understand and remember what you are reading.

Example 2–3 ————————————————————————

Read the following example from the Flynn health care textbook *Procedures in Phlebotomy*, (p. 126) and pay attention to the boldface directional words. Focus on the order of the information presented. Count the number of steps in the procedure.

SYRINGE COLLECTIONS

Because blood will begin to clot in the syringe, it is imperative that collected blood be added to the anticoagulant tubes, **first** starting with yellow-stoppered tubes (for blood cultures), **followed** by any other anticoagulant tubes, and **then** any remaining tubes without anticoagulant. The phlebotomist should mix the anticoagulant tubes thoroughly **after** the blood has been added.

EXERCISE 2–3

Directions: Read the following selection from a health care textbook (Young and Kennedy, p. 273). Then answer the questions that follow.

Preparing Monthly Billing Statements

Goal: To process monthly statements and evaluate accounts for collection procedures in accordance with the agency's credit policy.

EQUIPMENT AND SUPPLIES

- Typewriter or computer
- Patient accounts
- Agency's credit policy
- Statement forms

PROCEDURAL STEPS

1. Assemble all accounts that have outstanding balances.
2. Separate accounts that need special attention in accordance with the agency's credit policy.
   Explanation: Routine statements should be prepared first, after which special attention can be given to delinquent accounts.
3. Prepare routine statements, including the following:

   - Date the statement is prepared
   - Name and address of the person responsible for payment
   - Name of the patient, if different from the person responsible for payment
   - Itemization of dates, services, and charges for the month
   - Any unpaid balance carried forward (may or may not be itemized, depending on office policy)

4. Determine the action to be taken on accounts separated in Step 2.
5. Make a note of the necessary action on the ledger card (telephone call, collection letter series, small claims court, or assignment of collection agency).
   Purpose: To be used for guidance in executing an action and for later follow-up when necessary.

1. The selection is mainly about <u>MONTHLY BILLING STATEMENTS</u>
2. How many steps must be followed to complete the directions? <u>5</u>
3. List the directional words that lead you to each step. <u>1st, after, later</u>
4. Look at this scrambled list of steps from the reading selection. Rearrange the steps in the correct order. Number the steps in their proper order.

   <u>1</u> Assemble all accounts that have oustanding balances.

   <u>4</u> Determine the action to be taken on separate accounts that need special attention.

   <u>5</u> Make a note of the necessary action on a ledger card.

   <u>3</u> Prepare routine statements.

   <u>2</u> Separate accounts that need special attention.

Sequence

The sequence pattern helps you to understand a process when you read your health care textbook. Sequence helps you to answer these questions about any procedure:

What does it do? How does it work? You answer these questions by following an order or sequence. This helps you to organize the information into a system. Some signal words that help you to follow a sequence pattern are *steps, when, then, first, last, stages.* Following a sequence helps you understand each step of any procedure described in your textbook.

Example 2–4

Read the following example of a sequence pattern of organization from the Chabner textbook *The Language of Medicine*, (p. 413). Notice how the signal words **after, initial, and second** help you to follow the process of digital subtraction angiography (DSA).

DIGITAL SUBTRACTION ANGIOGRAPHY (DSA)

Video equipment and a computer produce x-ray images of blood vessels. After taking an initial x-ray and storing it in a computer, physicians inject contrast material and take a second image of that area. The computer compares the two images and subtracts the first from the second, leaving an image of vessels with contrast.

EXERCISE 2–4

Directions: Read the following excerpt from a health care textbook (Bird and Robinson, pp. 762 and 763). Follow the pattern of organization. Answer the questions following the selection.

MIXING A TWO-PASTE FINAL IMPRESSION MATERIAL
Equipment and Supplies

- Stock or custom tray with appropriate adhesive
- Large, stiff, tapered spatulas (2)
- Large paper pads (2)
- Light-bodied base and catalyst
- Heavy-bodied base and catalyst
- Impression syringe with sterile tip
- 2- × 2-inch gauze pads

Procedural Steps
Preparing Light-Bodied Syringe Material

1. Dispense approximately $1^1/2$ to 2 inches of equal lengths of the base and catalyst of the light-bodied material onto the top third of the pad, making sure that the materials are not too close to each other.
   Purpose: Some paste materials tend to start spreading on the pad, and it is important to prevent a premature reaction.
2. Wipe the tube openings clean with gauze; recap immediately.
   Purpose: Cleaning the top of the tube and the threads prevents the cap from becoming messy and sticking.
3. Place the tip of the spatula blade into the catalyst and base; then mix in a swirling direction for approximately 5 seconds.

4. Gather the material onto the flat portion of the spatula. Place it on a clean area of the pad, preferably the center.
   Purpose: By beginning the mix on a clean area of the pad, you will obtain a more homogenous mix.
5. Spatulate smoothly, wiping back and forth and trying to use only one side of the spatula during the mixing process.
   Purpose: Material is lost by using both sides of the blade.
6. To obtain a more homogeneous mix, pick the material up by the spatula blade and wipe it onto the pad.
   Purpose: To pull the material from the bottom to the top of the mix.
7. Gather the material together and take your syringe tube and begin "cookie cutting" the material into the syringe. Insert the plunger and express a small amount of the material to make sure it is in working order.
8. Transfer the syringe to the dentist, making sure the tip of the syringe is directed toward the tooth.

PREPARING HEAVY-BODIED TRAY MATERIAL

1. Dispense approximately 3 to 4 inches of equal lengths of the base and catalyst of the heavy-bodied material on the top third of the pad for a quadrant tray.
   Note: The amount of material placed depends on whether you are using a quadrant tray or a full-arch tray.
2. Place the tip of the spatula blade into the catalyst and base; then mix in a swirling direction for approximately 5 seconds.
3. Gather the material onto the flat portion of the spatula and place it on a clean area of the pad, preferably the center.
   Purpose: Starting the mix on a clean area of the pad results in a more homogeneous mix.
4. Spatulate smoothly, wiping back and forth and trying to use only one side of the spatula during the mixing process.
   Purpose: Material is lost by using both sides of the blade.
5. To get a more homogeneous mix, pick the material up by the spatula blade and wipe it on the pad.
   Purpose: To pull the material from the bottom to the top of the mix.
6. Gather the bulk of the material with the spatula and load it into the tray. The best way to complete this without incorporating air is to use the flat side of the spatula and follow around the outside rim of the tray, "wiping" the material into the tray.
7. Using the tip of the spatula, spread the material evenly from one end of the tray to the other without picking up the material.
   Purpose: When you pull the material in an upward direction, you are incorporating air into the mixture.
8. Retrieve the syringe from the dentist and transfer the tray, making sure the dentist is able to grasp the handle of the tray properly.

1. What is the pattern of organization? _Sequence_
2. What is the topic? _MIXING A 2-PASTE FINAL IMPRESSION MATERIAL_
3. How many steps are in the first procedure? _8_
4. Number these steps in the order in which they take place in the procedure.

    _3_ Place the blade of the spatula into the catalyst and base.

    _1_ Dispense syringe-type materials onto a clean paper pad.

_5_ Transfer the syringe to the dentist.

_2_ Wipe the tube openings clean with gauze.

_4_ Spatulate smoothly.

Classification

The classification pattern is used to group and subgroup the different facts in your text. Classification helps you to understand structure. By following classification patterns, you will be able to understand **how things are organized, how things are made,** and **what things are.** Classification is also used to describe things. Charts are often used to illustrate this pattern. Some signal words that are clues to recognizing this pattern are _breaks down, parts, components, group, heading,_ and _subheading._ When you recognize and follow the classification pattern in your health care texts, you will be able to find the more important and less important details. Therefore, you will be able to understand the content of your reading assignment.

Example 2–5 ──────────────────────

Read the following example of a **classification** pattern from Chabner (pp. 566-567). Follow the organization of details. See how the relationship between the six parts and the whole (facial bones) help you to understand the content. Examine how labeling the parts of the diagram will help you to understand and remember the information in the selection.

FACIAL BONES

All the facial bones, except one, are joined together by sutures, so that they are immovable. The mandible (lower jaw bone) is the only facial bone capable of movement. This ability is necessary for activities such as mastication (chewing) and speaking.

Figure 2-1 shows the facial bones; label it as you read the following descriptions of the facial bones:

(1) **Nasal bones**—Two slender nasal (**nas/o** means nose) bones support the bridge of the nose. They join with the frontal bone superiorly and form part of the nasal septum.

(2) **Lacrimal bones**—Two paired lacrimal (**lacrim/o** means tear) bones are located at the corner of each eye. These thin, small bones contain fossae for the lacrimal gland (tear gland) and canals for the passage of the lacrimal duct.

(3) **Maxillary bones**—Two large bones compose the massive upper jawbones (**maxillae**). They are joined by a suture in the median plane. If the two bones do not come together normally before birth, the condition know as **cleft palate** results.

(4) **Mandibular bone**—This is the lower jawbone (**mandible**). Both the maxilla and the mandible contain the sockets called **alveoli** in which the teeth are embedded. The mandible joins the skull at the region of the temporal bone, forming the temporo-mandibular joint (TMJ) on either side of the skull.

(5) **Zygomatic bones**—Two bones, one on each side of the face, form the high portion of the cheek.

(6) **Vomer**—This thin, single, flat bone forms the lower portion of the nasal septum.

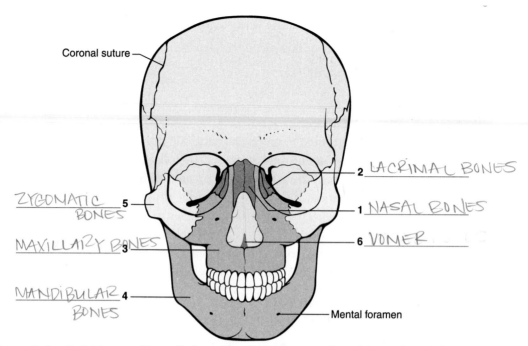

Coronal suture

2 LACRIMAL BONES

ZYGOMATIC 5
BONES

1 NASAL BONES

MAXILLARY BONES 3

6 VOMER

MANDIBULAR 4
BONES

Mental foramen

FIGURE 2–1 Facial bones. (From Chabner DE: The Language of Medicine, ed 7, Philadelphia, WB Saunders, 2004, p. 567.)

EXERCISE 2–5

Directions: Read the following textbook selection (Chabner, p. 47). Answer the questions based on the selection. Identify the pattern of organization. Use this pattern to help you understand the passage.

QUADRANTS

The abdominopelvic area can be divided into four quadrants by drawing two imaginary lines—one horizontally and one vertically through the body. Figure 2-2 shows these quadrants. You add the proper abbreviation under each label on the diagram.

Right upper quadrant (RUQ) contains the liver (right lobe), gallbladder, part of the pancreas, parts of the small and large intestines.

Left upper quadrant (LUQ) contains the liver (left lobe), stomach, spleen, part of the pancreas, parts of the small and large intestines.

Right lower quadrant (RLQ) contains parts of the small and large intestines, right ovary, right fallopian tube, appendix, right ureter.

Left lower quadrant (LLQ) contains parts of the small and large intestines, left ovary, left fallopian tube, left ureter.

1. What is the pattern of organization? CLASSIFICATION

2. Did you add the abbreviations under each label?

    Yes_____YES_____

    No_____

3. What is the main topic? ____QUADRANTS____

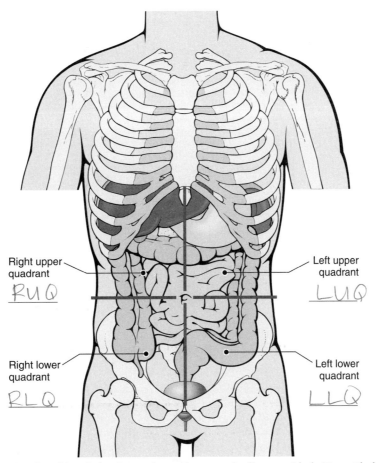

FIGURE 2–2 Give the abbreviation for each quadrant on the line provided. (From Chabner DE: The Language of Medicine, ed 7, Philadelphia, WB Saunders, 2004, p. 47.)

Right upper quadrant   *RUQ*
Left upper quadrant   *LUQ*
Right lower quadrant   *RLQ*
Left lower quadrant   *LLQ*

4. How many parts are there? ___*4*___
5. List the parts: *RUQ, RLQ, LUQ, LLQ* _____
   _____
6. Which part contains the gallbladder? *RUQ* _____

EXERCISE 2–6

Directions: Read the following excerpt from a health care textbook (Chabner, pp. 48-49). Follow the pattern of organization. Answer the questions following the selection.

DIVISIONS OF THE BACK (SPINAL COLUMN)

The spinal column is composed of a series of bones extending from the neck to the tailbone. Each bone is called a **vertebra** (plural: **vertebrae**).

Label the divisions of the back on Figure 2-3 as you study the following:

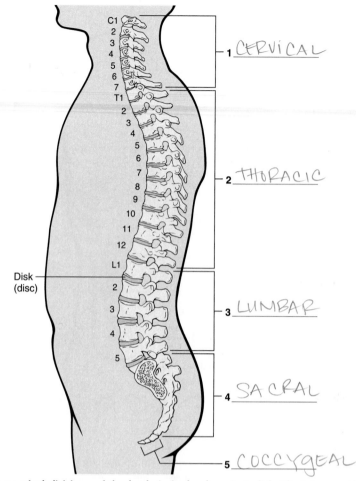

FIGURE 2–3 Anatomical divisions of the back (spinal column). A disk (disc) is a small pad of cartilage between each backbone (vertebra). (From Chabner DE: The Language of Medicine, ed 7, Philadelphia, WB Saunders, 2004, p. 48.)

DIVISION OF THE BACK	ABBREVIATION	LOCATION
(1) Cervical	C	Neck region. There are seven cervical vertebrae (C1-C7).
(2) Thoracic	T	Chest region. There are twelve thoracic vertebrae (T1-T12). Each bone is joined to a rib.
(3) Lumbar	L	Loin (waist) or flank region (between the ribs and the hipbone). There are five lumbar vertebrae (L1-L5).
(4) Sacral	S	Five bones (S1-S5) are fused to form one bone, the **sacrum**.
(5) Coccygeal		The **coccyx** (tailbone) is a small bone composed of four fused pieces.

1. What is the pattern of organization? _CLASSIFICATION_
2. Did you label each part?

   Yes _YES_   No _____
3. What is the main topic? _DIVISIONS OF THE BACK_
4. Write the number of the part that contains the neck region. ___1_____
5. Write the number of the part that contains the chest region. ___2_____

Examples and Illustrations

When you read health care textbooks, the author may give examples or illustrations as the details to back up his main ideas. Signal words that are a clue to this pattern are *for example*, *shows*, *explains*, *kinds of*. Following these examples will help you to understand the ideas in your text.

Example 2–6

Read the following example of an **examples or illustrations** pattern (Bird and Robinson, p. 739). The signal words, *three ways*, gives you a clue to follow examples. Read and follow these types of dental cement. Look at Figure 2-4 to see how these types of dental cement are used.

DENTAL BASES

When a posterior tooth ends up becoming a moderately deep to deep preparation, the dentist will most likely choose to place a base under the permanent restoration. A base is an additional layer in the restoration process in order to protect the pulp. A base is designed to provide pulpal protection in the following three ways:

1. *Protective bases* are placed when it is necessary to protect the pulp before the restoration is placed. Without this protection, there may be postoperative sensitivity and damage to the pulp.
2. *Insulating bases* are placed in a deep cavity preparation to protect the tooth from thermal shock. (*Thermal shock* occurs when sudden temperature changes occur within the tooth).
3. *Sedative bases* help soothe a pulp that has been damaged by decay or has been irritated during the process of removing the decay.

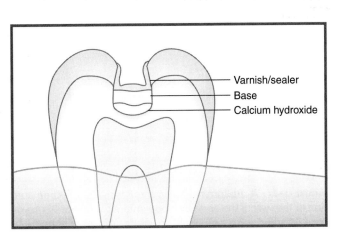

FIGURE 2–4   Location for placement of base. (From Bird DL, Robinson DS: Torres and Ehrlich Modern Dental Assisting, ed 8, Philadelphia, Saunders, 2005, p. 731)

EXERCISE 2-7

Directions: Read the following excerpt from a health care textbook (Chabner, p. 408). Follow the pattern of organization. Answer the questions following the selection.

An **aneurysm** (Greek, *aneurysma*, widening) is usually caused by atherosclerosis and hypertension or a congenital weakness in the vessel wall. Aneurysms are common in the aorta, but may occur in peripheral vessels as well. The danger of an aneurysm is rupture and hemorrhage. Treatment depends on the vessel involved, the site, and the health of the patient. In aneurysms of small vessels in the brain (**berry aneurysms**), treatment is occlusion of the vessel with small clips. For larger arteries, such as the aorta, the aneurysm is resected and a synthetic graft is sewn within the aneurysm. Figure 2-5A shows an abdominal aortic aneurysm, and Figure 2-5B illustrates a synthetic graft in place. Stent grafts may also be placed less invasively as an alternative to surgery in some patients.

HYPERTENSION (HTN)

High blood pressure. Most high blood pressure is **essential hypertension**, with no identifiable cause. In adults, a blood pressure equal to or greater than 140/90 mm Hg is considered high. Diuretics, beta-blockers, ACE inhibitors, and calcium channel blockers are used as treatment for essential hypertension. Losing weight, limiting **sodium** (salt) intake, stopping smoking, and reducing fat in the diet can reduce hypertension.

In **secondary hypertension**, the HTN is caused by another associated lesion, such as glomerulonephritis, pyelonephritis, or disease of the adrenal glands.

1. What is the pattern of organization? <u>EXAMPLES AND ILLUSTRATION</u>
2. What is the topic? <u>HIGH BLOOD PRESSURE IN ARTERIES</u>
3. What was given as an example of high blood pressure in adults? <u>=> 140/90 MM HG IS TOO HIGH</u>
4. What are treatments for hypertension? _____
5. What are the two kinds of hypertension? <u>ESSENTIAL AND SECONDARY.</u>

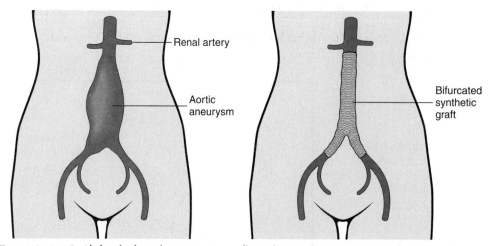

Renal artery

Aortic aneurysm

Bifurcated synthetic graft

FIGURE 2-5   A, Abdominal aortic aneurysm. A dissecting aortic aneurysm is splitting or dissection of the wall of the aorta by blood entering a tear or hemorrhage within the walls of the vessel. **B,** Bifurcated synthetic graft in place. (From Chabner DE: The Language of Medicine, ed 7, Philadelphia, WB Saunders, 2004, p. 409.)

Comparison and Contrast

Writers often organize details to compare or contrast information. Some signal words that help you to make comparisons are *alike, some, similar,* or *compare.* Some signal words that help you to contrast details are *different, other, unlike.* Comparison-contrast patterns help you to organize information so that you will remember which details are the same and which are different.

Example 2–7

Read the following example of a comparison-contrast pattern from Young and Kennedy (p. 5). The words *some* and *other* are signals to compare/contrast the organization of the details. Read about the differences between concrete and abstract perceivers. Use comparison and contrast to help you determine which way you perceive new material.

Information perception involves how you go about examining new material and making it real. There are two ways learners perceive new material. Some people are concrete perceivers who learn information through direct experience by doing, acting, sensing, or feeling. *Concrete* learners prefer to learn things that have a personal meaning or things that they feel are relevant. Other learners are *abstract* perceivers who take in information through analysis, observation, and **reflection**. Abstract learners like to think things through. They analyze the new material and build theories to help understand it. They prefer structured learning situations and use a step-by-step approach to problem solving.

EXERCISE 2–8

Directions: Read the following excerpt from the Purtilo health care textbook *Ethical Dimensions in the Health Professions,* (p. 191). Follow the pattern of organization. Answer the questions following the selections.

ARGUMENTS AGAINST DISCLOSURE

The main argument advanced against disclosure of "bad news" is that the health professional role is to maintain the patient's hope, and hope may be shattered by bad news. That may be what Maria's daughter was concerned about, and often health professionals have the same thoughts.

Throughout most of the history of Western health care the patient has been defined as the one who needs to be cared for, who has little knowledge of medical science, who suffers passively from a disease, and who brings herself or himself to the health care system much in the same way that a car is brought to an automobile mechanic. As Edward said to Dr. Reilly in T.S. Eliot's *The Cocktail Party,*

I can no longer act for myself.
Coming to see you—That's the last decision.
I was capable of making. I am in your hands.
I cannot take any further responsibility.

Both character traits and duties are involved in this type of professional-patient encounter. A professional's *benevolent disposition* has been regarded as more important than an honest one, although both are extremely important. Duties involved in this type of situation include beneficence, nonmaleficence, and veracity.

Arguments against disclosure of sensitive information have been based on paternalistic thinking. The health professional is privy to the awful truth of the inexorable progress of most diseases and decides what patients ought to be told based on an assessment of their welfare. Of course, such perceptions are heavily influenced by the professional's own concept of his or her role in the situation and attitudes about sickness and death.

This portrays a relationship that is unequal but well intentioned. Honesty is sacrificed to benevolence to maintain a patient's trust. As you can easily discern, Dr. Hammill is being benevolent insofar as he judges his course of action to be in Maria Priley's best interests. Now Kim Segard must make her own judgment about whether to act paternalistically or truthfully.

ARGUMENTS FAVORING DISCLOSURE

Today there is pressure on the health professions from within their own ranks (as well as from laypeople) to be candid and honest with patients. In the 1960s, Elisabeth Kübler-Ross, a physician, spearheaded a revolutionary movement in health care by clarifying simple concepts about the dying process and making suggestions to improve care of the dying. She was convinced that patients with fatal illnesses could handle the truth about that awesome knowledge, and therefore information ought not be swept under the rug delicately but rather dealt with honestly, carefully, and realistically. She cited many cases of people having come to terms with the meaning of death and dying for themselves and their loved ones because they knew the truth about their own condition and its prognosis. Currently, thanks to Kübler-Ross and others like her, the topics of dying and death are not as taboo as they were a few years ago, but also there is a new openness in communication about many kinds of sensitive information. The idea that patients can handle difficult news, and may even benefit from knowing, has taken the health professionals down a new line of reasoning: the truth, rather than being a barrier to hope, may set the patient free. The AIDS epidemic has raised truth-telling questions and concerns to the forefront of health professionals' consciousness, because if the patient does not know, he or she cannot be responsible for preventing the spread of the disease.

In this interpretation an honest disposition is at least as important as, and is not necessarily in conflict with, a benevolent one. Acting truthfully is consistent with acting beneficently. You cannot discern what is "best" for the patient by making decisions independently on his or her behalf. Caring entails sharing pertinent information. The best way to maintain trust is to share relevant information with patients but to do so in ways that will be supportive of them.

Underlying this bias toward greater disclosure of information is the conviction that if you convey the message that you still care and have the intention and ability to comfort, then it is possible to tell the truth and still maintain the patient's trust and hope. Benevolence is expressed *through* honesty rather than played off *against* it.

1. What is the pattern of organization? COMPARISON-CONTRAST
2. What is the topic? DISCLOSURE VS. ARGUMENTS
3. List the three details for disclosure. HONESTY, DEATH NOT TABOO, CARING ENTAILS
4. List the three details against disclosure. HOPE OF PT, PT PASSIVE, BENEVOLENCE
5. Which point of view do you agree with? _____ Why? _____

_____

_____

Cause and Effect

Cause-effect patterns of detail help you to answer the questions: *Why does it happen? How does it happen? How does it work?* Some signal words that help you to recognize cause-effect patterns are *because, in order to, why, result, effect, reasons, factors.* When following cause-effect patterns, remember that the cause takes place first; the effect happens after the cause.

Example 2–8

Read the following example of a **cause-effect** pattern of organization from Chabner (p. 406). Following this pattern will help you to understand **why** high blood pressure affects the heart.

HYPERTENSIVE HEART DISEASE

High blood pressure affecting the heart. This condition results from narrowing of arterioles, which leads to increased pressure in arteries. The heart is affected (left ventricular hypertrophy) because it pumps more vigorously to overcome the increased resistance in the arteries.

EXERCISE 2–9

Directions: Read the following excerpt from a health care textbook (Chabner, p. 403). Follow the pattern of organization. Answer the questions following the selection.

CONGESTIVE HEART FAILURE (CHF)

The heart is unable to pump its required amount of blood (more blood enters the heart from the veins than leaves through the arteries). Blood accumulates in the lungs (left-sided heart failure) causing **pulmonary edema** (fluid seeps out of capillaries into the tiny air sacs of the lungs). Damming back of blood resulting from right-sided heart failure results in accumulation of fluid in the abdominal organs (liver and spleen) and subcutaneous tissue of the legs. The most common cause of **CHF** in the United States is high blood pressure and coronary artery disease. Therapy includes lowering dietary intake of sodium and diuretics to promote loss of fluids.

Drugs (**angiotensin-converting enzyme [ACE] inhibitors** and **beta-blockers**) improve the performance of the heart and its pumping activity. These drugs decrease pressure inside blood vessels to treat hypertension (high blood pressure). If drug therapy and lifestyle changes fail to control congestive heart failure, heart transplantation may be the only treatment option. While waiting for a transplant, patients may need a device to assist the heart's pumping. A **left ventricular assist device (LVAD)** is a booster pump implanted in the abdomen, with a cannula (tube) inserted into the left ventricle. It pumps blood out of the heart to all parts of the body. The LVAD is sometimes called a "bridge to transplant."

1. What is the pattern of organization? _CAUSE-EFFECT_
2. What is the topic? _CONGESTIVE HEART FAILURE_
3. What is the reason for pulmonary edema? _HEART CAN'T PUMP REQ. AMOUNT OF BLOOD AND BLOOD ACCUMULATES TO LUNGS._
4. What gets into the lungs? _FLUID_
5. Why is there a damming back of blood? _RT. SIDE HEART FAILURE_

REVIEWING RECOGNIZING DETAILS

TO LEARN	USE THIS STRATEGY
To locate details	Locate the facts that give you a better understanding of the main idea
To distinguish between the main idea and important details	Remember that the main idea is a general statement and the details are specific facts

To map details	Recognize that there are important details which describe the main idea and less important details which describe the important details
To verify facts from the text	Scan for facts by focusing on key words to help you find the information you are looking for in the text
To recognize logical relationships	Recognize that main ideas and details are organized into types of patterns. Look for the following patterns in your textbook:

- Sequence
- Classification
- Examples and illustrations
- Comparison and contrast
- Cause and effect

Chapter 3

Developing Vocabulary

LEARNING OBJECTIVES

In this chapter you will learn how to
- Improve your general and medical vocabulary by learning strategies for using context clues, word parts, dictionaries, glossaries, and thesauruses
- Remember the meanings of new vocabulary terms by creating word cards

VOCABULARY WORDS

The following vocabulary words are important to your understanding of the ideas in this chapter. These vocabulary words are underscored the first time they are used in the chapter. Read the list of words and definitions. Then check your understanding of these words before you read the chapter.

analyzing breaking down a whole into its parts.

context the words around an unknown word that are used to figure out the meaning of the unknown word.

hormone a complex chemical substance produced in one part or organ of the body that initiates or regulates the activity of an organ or a group of cells in another part (Mosby's Dictionary, p. 901).

inadequate not good enough.

microorganisms organisms that are too small to be seen with the unaided eye.

ovum egg.

pathogenic having the ability to cause disease.

syllables parts of a word that contain at least one consonant and one vowel.

vague not clearly stated.

veterinary relating to the diagnosis and cure of disease in animals.

VOCABULARY CHECK

Directions: Choose the vocabulary word that best fits into the sentence.

1. The student figured out the meaning of "defibrillation" by looking at the _CONTEXT_ clue.

2. He did not understand what to do because her instructions were _VAGUE_.

3. _ANALYZING_ the parts of the plant was easy for the botany student.

4. Because of a _HORMONES_ imbalance, she was gaining much weight.

5. The small child was learning to read quickly by breaking up big words into _SYLLABLE_.

6. The doctor received an _INADEQUATE_ supply of the much needed drug.

7. The _VETERINARY_ surgeon operated on the dog.

8. In the laboratory, the scientists were looking at a human _OVUM_ in a test tube.

9. A _PATHOGENIC_ substance was released into the air causing thousands of people untold misery.

10. It is amazing that so many _MICROORG-ANISMS_ can be seen on the laboratory slide.

THE NEED FOR A GOOD VOCABULARY

Having chosen to become health care students, you have entered an environment where you will be exposed to new and unfamiliar words. You will come across these words in your textbooks, lectures, and conversations with instructors and fellow students. A great deal of your school success will depend on how many of these words you understand and on the strategies that you use to learn and remember words you do not know.

You will be expected to know two types of vocabulary words. The first type, general terminology, includes the words you hear around you every day or words that you see in newspapers, magazines, and books that you read for pleasure. The second type, medical terminology, includes the specific words that relate to your studies in the health care field. Different strategies are required to learn and remember these two types of vocabulary words. When you read or hear a general vocabulary term that you do not understand, it is sometimes okay not to know the exact or precise definition of the word. If you have a close enough understanding of the word, that may be good enough. It is important in some instances not to stop the flow of your reading or quit taking class notes to look up an unknown word. However, this is not the case for learning and remembering medical terminology. When you read or hear new medical terms in your textbook and lectures, it is very important to get the precise definitions of these words. Therefore, it is necessary not only to learn new words but also to choose the right strategies for learning general vocabulary and medical vocabulary words.

CONTEXT CLUES

An excellent strategy for learning both general and medical vocabulary words is using context clues. When you use context clues, you try to figure out the meaning of the unknown word by reading the surrounding words in the sentence or paragraph.

EXERCISE 3–1

Directions: Look at the following exercise from a passage in *Clinical Textbook for Veterinary Technicians,* by McCurnin (p. 27). Notice that some of the words have been left out. See if you can determine what words belong in the blanks by reading the surrounding words in the passage.

Most ~~CATHETER COATED~~ entering the field of veterinary medicine have had experience with some ~~OIL GLANDS~~, but few have had the experience necessary to deal with all ~~TAIL VEIN~~ that may be encountered. To assume all animals respond in the same manner is not correct and can be quite dangerous. Restraint ~~USED ONCE~~ differ markedly among species, and the responses of different animals to restraint are also highly variable.

After reading the entire passage you should have filled in "people," "animals," "species," and "techniques." What you have just done is use the surrounding and familiar words to figure out the unknown words. In other words, you have used context clues to fill in the blank spaces. The advantage to this strategy is that you do not have to stop reading to look up a word in the dictionary. Nor do you need to stop taking notes in a lecture class to get the definition of an unknown word. Using context clues, or the surrounding words, to figure out the meaning of an unknown word is a fine strategy for learning both general and medical vocabulary. However, some context clues will give you only a vague definition that may be acceptable for general vocabulary words and other context clues may give a precise definition that will work well with unknown medical words. It is your responsibility to be aware of when context clues are meeting your vocabulary needs, and when they are not you must use another strategy to learn the definition of the unknown word.

Locating Context Clues

To use context clues, you must be able to locate or recognize which words in the sentence or paragraph are suggesting the definition of the unknown word. Sometimes, the context clue will be right next to the unknown word, separated from it by a comma or a dash. Read the following example from *Health Unit Coordinating*, by LaFleur Brooks and Gillingham, (p. 20).

Example 3–1

A **radiologist**, a medical doctor qualified in the use of x-ray and other imaging devices, is in charge of this department.

Note that in this example, the definition "a medical doctor qualified in the use of x-ray and other imaging devices" is separated from the unknown medical term *radiologist* by commas. This context clue gives us a precise definition of the word *radiologist*.

EXERCISE 3–2

Directions: Read the following sentences and circle the context clue for the **boldfaced** word in each sentence.

1. **Radiopaque catheter** a catheter coated with a substance that does not allow the passage of x-rays, thus allowing the movement of the catheter to be followed on the viewing screen (LaFleur Brooks and Gillingham, p. 313).
2. **Sebaceous glands** (see-bay'-shus), also known as *oil glands*, are generally attached to hair follicles (Solomon, p. 43).
3. The **ventral coccygeal vein**, on the ventral aspect of the tail, can be used as a site for injection of small volumes of medication. Because of the proximity of the coccygeal vein to the coccygeal artery and the fecal contamination around the tail, the vein is not recommended for injections (McCurnin, p. 126).
4. **Disposable** thermometers (those that are used only once) are also available for obtaining body temperatures (Young and Kennedy, p. 527).
5. **Kardex File** a portable file that contains and organizes by room number the **Kardex** forms for each patient on the nursing unit (LaFleur Brooks and Gillingham, p. 160).

Sometimes the context clue can be found in the same sentence as the unknown word. In this case, the context clue will appear as an exact definition of the unknown word. This type of context clue is frequently found in your health care textbooks. Look at this example of a context clue that appears in the same sentence as the unknown word.

Example 3–2

In an **ectopic (tubal) pregnancy,** the fertilized *ovum* is planted outside of the uterus; over 90% implant in the fallopian tubes (LaFleur Brooks and Gillingham, p. 558).

In this example, the words "*the fertilized ovum is planted outside of the uterus*" provide a clear and precise definition for the unknown medical term *ectopic pregnancy.*

EXERCISE 3–3

Directions: In the space provided, write a definition context clue for each of the following medical terms. Consult a dictionary if necessary but use your own words for writing the sentences. The first one has been done for you.

1. Crown: <u>The crown of the tooth is above the gumline.</u>
2. Insomnia: _____
3. Nausea: _____
4. Tonsillectomy: _____
5. Iris: _____
6. Estrogen: _____

In some instances, however, you may have to read an entire paragraph or a longer passage to find the context clues that suggest the meaning of an unknown word. This may be the case for both general and medical terms. Read the following selection from LaFleur-Brooks and Gillingham, (p. 508). Notice that the italicized context clues for "anemia" are found in the sentences following the boldfaced word **anemia.**

Example 3–3

Anemia is a disorder characterized by an abnormally low level of hemoglobin in the blood or inadequate numbers of RBCs. It may result from *decreased RBC production*, from *increased RBC destruction*, or from *blood loss*. Treatment varies according to the cause. The anemic person becomes easily fatigued. Pallor may also indicate anemia. Sternal puncture to obtain bone marrow for study and blood tests are used to diagnose anemia.

EXERCISE 3–4

Directions: Read the following passage from *The Medical Assistant; An Applied Learning Approach* by Young and Kennedy, (p. 73). Underline all the words that are context clues that help you figure out the meaning of the phrase *subtle discrimination.*

Discrimination is a word that is used to describe unfair treatment of a person because of race, gender, religious affiliation, handicap, or any other reason. Discrimination is unethical, morally and socially wrong, and in many situations, it is illegal. It also prevents us from communicating effectively.

Some discriminaton is very **subtle**; it is not expressed openly or in a blatant manner. Subtle discrimination is based on a person's appearance, values, lifestyle, or some other personal factor. Examples include discrimination against those who are obese, divorced individuals, homosexuals, welfare recipients, or those with sexually transmitted diseases.

Sometimes we are not aware that our words or actions reflect subtle discrimination against others.

WORD PARTS

Another good strategy for learning unknown words is analyzing the meaning of the word parts that make up the structure of the word. This strategy can be used for general vocabulary, but it is particularly effective for medical terms as long as these words have word parts. By learning and remembering a relatively small number of word parts, you will be able to discover the meanings of thousands of unknown words.

What Are Word Parts?

Many medical and general words in English are made up of two or more of the following word parts:

A **prefix** is a word part that is found in the beginning of the word. It changes the meaning of the main part of the word. For example, when you add the prefix *un* to the main part of the word *happy,* the meaning changes from "glad" to "not being glad."

A **root** is a word part that is the main part of the word and gives the basic meaning to the word. For example, in the word *review, view* is the root and means "to see." When you add the prefix *re,* the meaning of the root changes and the word now means "to see again."

A **suffix** is a word part that is found at the end of the word. It has two purposes. The first purpose is to change the meaning of the root. The second purpose is to change the part of speech. For example, in the medical word *endocrinologist,* the suffix *ologist* means "a person who studies." This suffix changes the meaning of the root *crin* ("to give off") to "one who studies that which is given off." The suffix changes the root from a verb (action word) to a noun (person, place, or thing). When you add the prefix *endo* ("within"), you now see that the word *endocrinologist* means "one who studies that which gives off from within." This refers to the various glands that secrete, or give off, hormones. Thus an endocrinologist is a person who specializes in the study of the function and disorders of the glands that give off hormones.

You can see from this example that when you know the meanings of some prefixes, roots, and suffixes you will be able to use your knowledge to analyze word parts to determine the meanings of many unknown words. However, you must be aware that in some cases a word may seem to have a word part but that word part may really be the root and cannot be used to figure out the meaning of the word. For example, the word *reptile* may appear to begin with the prefix *re,* but that is just a part of the root. Thus when you try to use the word part strategy, be sure that the word part is indeed a word part. To do this, familiarize yourself with some of the word parts and their meanings in Table 3-1.

EXERCISE 3–5

Directions: In Table 3-1 in the column headed "Definition of Example," write the meanings of the example words for prefixes, roots, and suffixes. Check with a dictionary or glossary if necessary.

TABLE 3–1 Prefixes, Roots, Suffixes

Prefix	Definition	Example	Definition of Example	Your Example
anti	against	anti-inflammatory		
*dys	bad, difficult	dyslexia		
*exo	outside	exoskeleton		
*hyper	over, above, beyond	hyperkinesias		
inter	between	intersession		
mal	poor, bad	maladjusted		
*peri	around, near	perigastric		
semi	half	semisweet		
tele	distant, far	telescope		
Root				
*arthro, arthr	joint	arthritis		
bio	life	biology		
*cardi, cardio	heart	cardiopathy		
*derm dermo	skin	dermatitis		
fac, fact	make, do	factory		
*hem, hemato	relating to the blood	hemodiagnosis		
*path	disease	pathologist		
port	carry	portable		
*psych	mind	psychiatry		
spec, spect	to look at	spectator		
vers	turn	reversible		
Suffix				
able, ible	capable of	trainable		
ation	act of	sanitation		
*ectomy	excision	hysterectomy		
ful	full of	hateful		
*itis	inflammation	bursitis		
ology	study of	psychology		
*oma	tumor	hematoma		
*osis	condition	nephrosis		
*phobia	fear	xenophobia		
scope	see	periscope		

*Word parts with a medical use.

EXERCISE 3–6

Directions: In the column headed "Your Example," write your own example word for each prefix, root, and suffix. If necessary, use a dictionary, glossary, or thesaurus.

EXERCISE 3–7

Directions: Make up your own chart similar to the one in Table 3-1. Write in any prefixes, roots, and suffixes you see in your textbook and would like to learn.

THE DICTIONARY, GLOSSARY, AND THESAURUS

In this chapter, you have learned vocabulary development strategies that allow you to continue reading your textbook if you see a word you do not understand. However, you may discover that not all sentences and paragraphs contain context clues and not all words are made up of word parts. In that case, you will have to stop the flow of your reading and consult with a reference that will give you the definition. Also, when you are working with medical terminology, it is important to know the precise definition of the word. Then, again, it will be necessary to consult a dictionary, glossary, or thesaurus for help in finding the meaning of the unknown word.

The Dictionary

As a health care student, it will be necessary for you to own two types of dictionaries; a **collegiate** dictionary for learning general vocabulary and a **medical** dictionary for learning medical terms. You may find it convenient to own two versions of a collegiate dictionary—a hard-cover version to keep at home by your study area and a softcover version to carry to school.

Many students do not realize that a dictionary contains more than just definitions. A good dictionary will show you how to pronounce a word, the origin of the word, how to break the word into syllables, and other words that mean the same or the opposite of the word you are looking up.

Reading a Dictionary Entry

To be able to use the dictionary well, you must be familiar with the various parts of the entry. Following is an entry taken from *Mosby's Dictionary*, (p. 1188). The different parts of the entry have been numbered.

1.   2.   3.   4.   5.

metastasis (me-tas´tah-sis), *pl. metastases* [Gk, *meta* + *stasis*, standing], 1. the process by which tumor cells spread to distant parts of the body. Because malignant tumors have no enclosing capsule, cells may escape, become emboli, and be transported by the lymphatic circulation or the bloodstream to implant in lymph nodes and other organs far from the primary tumor. 2. a tumor that develops away from the site of origin.

6.   7.

Compare **anaplasia.** –**metastatic,** *adj.*, **metastasize,** *v.*

Let us look closer at the different numbered parts of the entry:

1. The **main entry** or **headword** is printed in boldface type. This is the word you are looking up.
2. The **pronunciation** is found next to the headword and is enclosed in parentheses ( ). The headword is broken into syllables using dashes and written with accent marks to help you pronounce the word.
3. The **plural** form of the headword is given if it is not a standard English plural.
4. The **derivation** or **origin** of the word is given if the word comes from a foreign country. The derivation is abbreviated, and the meaning of the abbreviation can be found in the beginning of the dictionary.
5. The **definitions** or **meanings** of the headword follow and are printed in regular type. If there is more than one meaning for the word, the definitions will be numbered. When you are looking up an unknown word, it is important that you choose the definition that fits into the context of what you are reading.
6. **Cross References,** preceded by "see also" or "compare" refer to another defined entry for additional information.
7. The **adjective** or **verb form** of the headword is also provided, if there is one. It is printed in boldface and broken up into its pronunciation.

EXERCISE 3–8

Directions: Reread the dictionary entry at the top of this page and answer the following questions in the space provided.

1. The headword is ___METASIS___
2. How is the headword printed? ___BOLD FACE___
3. How many syllables are in the headword? ___FOUR___
4. The headword comes from what foreign country? ___GREECE___
5. If you were reading about a cancerous tumor spreading from the breast to the brain, which numbered definition would be best? ___ONE___
6. Into what other part of speech can the headword be changed? ___ADJ. VERB___
7. What is a synonym for the headword? ___ANAPLASIA___

The Glossary

The glossary is a listing of key words found in the back of some of your textbooks. A glossary is like a dictionary because it gives you the definitions of words. However, the entries in a glossary are much briefer than dictionary entries. A glossary entry usually omits pronunciation, plural form, derivation, adjective form, and synonyms. It is generally just a collection of important words from the textbook and their definitions.

The advantage of the glossary is its convenience. You do not need to put down your textbook and start searching for a dictionary. The words are found in the back of the text you are reading. The disadvantage of the glossary is its limited number of words. You may discover that a needed word is not listed in the glossary. Only words that the author believes are important are included in the glossary. A word that you believe is important or do not know may not be included. Also, the glossary entry, as mentioned earlier, is much briefer than an entry in the dictionary, so you will not learn all you can about an unknown word. In any case, if you need to know the exact definition of a medical term, the glossary can be the first place you look. If the information is <u>inadequate,</u> use your medical dictionary.

EXERCISE 3–9

Directions: The first page of a glossary taken from the Solomon health-care textbook *Introduction to Human Anatomy and Physiology,* (p. 293) is shown on p. 47. Study the page and then answer the following questions in the space provided.

1. How many glands make up the adrenal glands? __TWO__
2. The Adam's apple is enlarged by which hormone? __TESTERONE__
3. The Achilles' tendon is attached to which bone? __HEEL BONE__
4. AIDS is an abbreviation for __ACQUIRED IMMUNE DEFICIENCY SYNDROME__
5. The area of the body between the diaphragm and the pelvis is the __ABDOMEN__ .

The Thesaurus

A thesaurus is a listing of words and their synonyms (different words that have the same meaning). In addition, some thesauruses will give words that mean the opposite of the headword (antonyms). Most thesauruses resemble a dictionary; you look up the entry the same way you would look up an entry in your dictionary. However, instead of giving pronunciations, origins, and definitions, a thesaurus lists only the words that can be used to substitute for the headword.

The thesaurus is most useful for good writing. When you are writing a paper, you may see that you are using the same word repeatedly. If this is so, look up the word in the thesaurus and choose a different word with the same meaning. Or else, you may want to use a word that has a different meaning than the word you have written. Again, consult the thesaurus. Once you become familiar with the thesaurus and use it regularly, you should notice a big improvement in your writing.

Reading a Thesaurus Entry

Following is an entry taken from *Roget's New Pocket Thesaurus in Dictionary Form* (p. 309). The different parts of the entry have been numbered.

1.	2.	3.	4.

physician, n. general practitioner, doctor (MEDICAL SCIENCE)

1. The **main entry** or **headword** is the word you are looking up in order to find a synonym for it.

GLOSSARY

■ ■ ■

abdomen (**ab′**-doe-men) The region of the body between the diaphragm and the pelvis.

abdominal (ab-**dom′**-ih-nal) **cavity** The superior part of the abdominopelvic cavity containing the liver, gallbladder, spleen, stomach, pancreas, small intestine, and part of the large intestine.

abdominopelvic (ab-dom′-ih-no-**pel′**-vic) **cavity** The lower part of the ventral body cavity below the thoracic cavity.

abduction (ab-**duk′**-shun) A movement whereby a body part is drawn away from the main body axis or the axis of a limb.

ABO blood types A system of categorizing blood, based on the presence or absence of specific antigens on the plasma membranes of red blood cells.

abortion (ah-**bor′**-shun) Expulsion of an embryo or fetus before it is capable of surviving outside the uterus.

absorption (ab-**sorp′**-shun) The passage of material into or through a cell or tissue, as in the movement of digested nutrients from the gastrointestinal (GI) tract into the blood or lymph.

accommodation The ability to change the curvature of the lens to clearly focus on objects at various distances.

acetylcholine (as′-eh-til-**koe′**-leen) A neurotransmitter released by cholinergic nerves, such as those stimulating skeletal muscle contraction.

Achilles′ (ah-**kil′**-eez) **tendon** The tendon of the gastrocnemius and soleus muscle that inserts upon the calcaneus (heel bone).

acid (**as′**-id) A substance that is a hydrogen ion (proton) donor; dissociates in solution to produce hydrogen ions and some type of anion.

acquired immunodeficiency syndrome (AIDS) A serious disease caused by the human immunodeficiency virus (HIV) in which a deficiency develops in helper T cells.

acromegaly (ak′-roe-**meg′**-ah-lee) A condition resulting from hypersecretion of growth hormone in the adult; characterized by enlarged bones in the extremities and face along with the enlargement of other tissues.

actin (**ak′**-tin) A contractile protein found in the thin filaments within a muscle cell.

actin filaments Thin filaments composed mainly of the protein *actin;* actin and myosin filaments make up the myofibrils of muscle fibers.

action potential An electrical signal that results from depolarization of the plasma membrane in a neuron or muscle cell; also called a *nerve* or *muscle impulse.*

active immunity An acquired immunity resulting from the production of antibodies in response to exposure to antigens.

active transport The movement of substances through cell membranes against concentration gradients. Active transport requires energy expenditure.

acute (a-**kyout′**) Having a short and relatively severe course; not chronic.

Adam's apple The thyroid cartilage of the larynx. In males, it is pronounced because of enlargement caused by testosterone.

adduction (ad-**duk′**-shun) A movement whereby a body part is drawn toward the main body axis or the axis of a limb.

adenosine triphosphate (a-**den′**-oh-seen try-**fos′**-fate) **(ATP)** See *ATP.*

adipose tissue A type of connective tissue in which fat is stored.

adrenal cortex (ah-**dree′**-nal **kore′**-tekz) The outer part of the adrenal gland; it has three zones, each producing different hormones.

adrenal (ah-**dree′**-nal) **glands** Paired endocrine glands, one located just superior to each kidney. They are also known as the *suprarenal glands.*

adrenal medulla (ah-**dree′**-nal meh-**dul′**-ah) The inner part of the adrenal gland that secretes catecholamines (epinephrine and norepinephrine) in response to sympathetic stimulation.

adrenergic (ad-ren-**er′**-jik) **neuron** A neuron that releases norepinephrine.

adrenocorticotropic (ad-ree′-no-kore-ti-kow-**trope′**-ik) **hormone (ACTH)** A hormone produced by

293

2. A letter **abbreviation** tells you **the part of speech** of the headword. An explanation of the abbreviations is usually given in the front of the thesaurus. Headwords may have more than one part of speech. Make sure that the part of speech matches the way the word appears in your text.

3. The **synonyms** are given following the part of speech.

4. Suggestions for **other words to look up** that relate to the word you want to change are written in capital letters, enclosed in parentheses, and end the entry.

EXERCISE 3–10

Page 192 from *Roget's New Pocket Thesaurus* is shown on p. 49. Read the following passage with words in boldface print. After reviewing the thesaurus page, choose a better word for each of the boldface words and write it above the boldface term. Make sure the part of speech of the synonym matches the part of speech of the word you want to change.

The **healer** wished to **heal** the patient with the bad heart. It was a **heartbreaking** situation because the patient came from a **heartless** family who did not care if she became **healthy** or not. They were very **headstrong** in their feelings. The family's attitude made the healer **heartsick**. If she could convince them that a change of heart would allow the patient to **heal** quicker, then she would feel **heartened** by the patient's improved ability to get **healthy**.

REMEMBERING NEW WORDS

In this chapter, you have learned different strategies for finding the meanings of unknown general and medical terms. However, seeing the definition of the unknown word is not the same as remembering the definition of the unknown word. You must have a strategy for memorizing the meaning of the word so you do not have to relearn the word every time you see it.

Word Cards

An excellent way of learning and retaining the meanings of new medical and general terms is to create word cards. To do this, you need to buy index cards that are lined on one side and blank on the other. On the blank side of the index card you write the unknown word. If you wish, you can copy the pronunciation of the word from the dictionary so you can remember how to say it at some later time. On the lined side of the index card, write the definition of the word. In addition, you may want to write a sentence with the word in it to help you remember how the word is actually used.

What you have now created with the index card is a flash card with which you can practice remembering the new word. Because the words are written on index cards, you can carry them anywhere and practice memorizing the words when it is convenient for you. Also, these words are words that you, rather than your instructor, have chosen to learn, so the memorizing process should be more meaningful for you. Finally, the cards are versatile, so you can use them in many ways. You may decide to look at the word and try to recall the definition. Or you may want to look at the definition and

HEADING 192 HEAT

mer (*slang*), derby, bowler (*Brit.*); castor, busby, cocked hat, coonskin hat, pith helmet, shako, sombrero, southwester *or* sou'-wester, tricorn; bonnet, capote, sunbonnet, calash, breton, cloche, picture hat, pillbox, sailor, toque.

cap, beanie, beret, biretta *or* barret (*R. C. Ch.*), coif, fez, tarboosh, garrison cap, overseas cap, kepi, mobcap, mob (*hist.*), mortarboard, nightcap, bedcap, skullcap, tam-o'-shanter, tam, tuque; cap and bells, fool's cap, dunce cap.

high hat, beaver, crush hat, opera hat, plug hat (*slang*), silk hat, stovepipe hat (*colloq.*), top hat, topper (*colloq.*).

helmet, headpiece, crest, casque (*poetic*); visor, beaver.

See also CLOTHING, CLOTHING WORKER, COVERING, HEAD, ORNAMENT. *Antonyms*—See FOOTWEAR.

heading, *n.* caption, rubric, inscription (TITLE).

headland, *n.* promontory, cape, head (LAND).

headline, *n.* banner, streamer, heading (TITLE).

headlong, *adv.* full-tilt, posthaste, pell-mell (SPEED); violently, headfirst, precipitately (VIOLENCE).

headstrong, *adj.* self-willed, obstinate, willful (STUBBORNNESS, WILL, UNRULINESS); ungovernable, uncontrollable, unruly (VIOLENCE).

headway, *n.* headroom, elbowroom, leeway, seaway (SPACE).

heady, *adj.* provocative, intoxicating, stimulating (EXCITEMENT).

heal, *v.* convalesce, mend, cure (HEALTH, CURE).

healer, *n.* medicine man, witch doctor, shaman (MEDICAL SCIENCE).

HEALTH—*N.* health, vigor, euphoria, eudaemonia, well-being; trim, bloom, pink, verdure, prime.

hygiene, sanitation, prophylaxis.

health resort, sanatorium, sanitarium, spa, watering place, rest home, convalescent home, hospital.

V. be in health, enjoy good health, bloom, flourish, thrive.

get well, convalesce, heal, mend, rally, recover, recuperate, revalesce, get better; cure, heal, restore to health, make well.

Adj. healthy, sound, well, robust, hearty, robustious (*jocose*), trim, trig, hale, fit, blooming, bouncing, strapping, vigorous, whole, wholesome, able-bodied, athletic, eudaemonic, euphoric, tonic.

convalescent, recovering, on the mend, recuperating, revalescent.

healthful, nutritious, salutary, salubrious, wholesome, beneficial; hygienic, sanatory, sanitary, prophylactic.

[*concerned about one's health*] hypochondriac, valetudinary, atrabilious.

unharmed, intact, untouched, scatheless, scot-free, sound, spared, unblemished, unbruised, undamaged, unhurt, uninjured, unmarred, unscarred, unscathed, unspoiled, unwounded, whole.

See also CURE, MEDICAL SCIENCE, RESTORATION, STRENGTH. *Antonyms*—See DISEASE.

heap, *n.* lump, pile, mass (ASSEMBLAGE).

heap up, *v.* pile up, stack, load (STORE).

hear, *v.* give a hearing to, overhear (LISTENING); try, sit in judgment (LAWSUIT).

hearing, *n.* audience, interview, conference (LISTENING); earshot, range (SOUND).

hearing aid, *n.* ear trumpet, auriphone, audiphone (LISTENING).

hearsay, *n.* comment, buzz, report (RUMOR).

heart, *n.* core, pith, kernel (CENTER, INTERIORITY); auricle, ventricle (BLOOD).

heartache, *n.* heavy heart, broken heart, heartbreak (SADNESS).

heartbreaking, *adj.* affecting, heart-rending, moving (PITY).

hearten, *v.* inspire, reassure, encourage (COURAGE).

heartfelt, *adj.* cordial, wholehearted (HONESTY).

hearth, *n.* fireplace, fireside, grate (HEAT); home, homestead, hearthstone (HABITATION).

heartless, *adj.* cruelhearted, flinthearted, hardhearted (CRUELTY); coldhearted, cold-blooded, cold (INSENSITIVITY).

heart-shaped, *adj.* cordiform, cordate (CURVE).

heartsick, *adj.* heartsore, heartstricken, heavyhearted (SADNESS).

hearty, *adj.* healthy, well, robust (HEALTH); cordial, sincere, glowing (FEELING).

HEAT—*N.* heat, warmth, temperature, calefaction, calescence, incalescence, candescence, incandescence.

[*instruments*] thermometer, calorimeter, pyrometer, centigrade *or* Celsius thermometer, Fahrenheit thermometer; thermostat, pyrostat, cryometer.

try to come up with the word. Whatever you decide, the use of the word cards allows you to be as creative as you wish in learning new medical and general vocabulary words.

EXERCISE 3–11

Directions: Using this textbook or any of your others, choose ten general vocabulary and ten medical vocabulary words and create word cards. Use Figure 3–1 as an example for setting up your cards. Use the two strategies suggested for memorizing the definitions, or invent your own strategies.

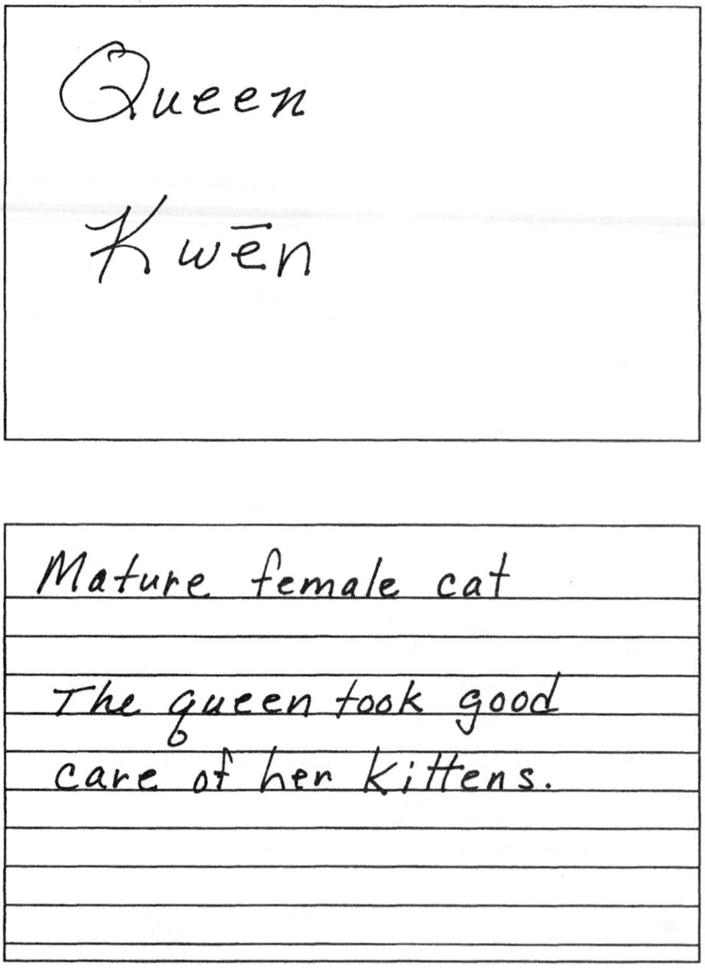

Queen

Kwēn

Mature female cat

The queen took good
care of her kittens.

FIGURE 3-1 Example of both sides of a word card.

REVIEWING THE LEARNING STRATEGIES

TO LEARN	USE THIS STRATEGY
To develop vocabulary	Context clues
	word parts
	dicitionaries
	glossaries
	thesauruses
To remember new vocabulary	word cards

Chapter 4

Monitoring and Improving Comprehension

LEARNING OBJECTIVES

In the chapter you will learn how to
- Become aware of when you do not understand what you are reading
- Use six strategies to improve comprehension

VOCABULARY WORDS

The following vocabulary words are important to your understanding of the ideas in this chapter. These vocabulary words are underscored the first time they are used in the chapter. Read the list of words and definitions. Then check your understanding of these words before you read the chapter.

approximate nearly the same or nearly correct.

attending physician a doctor who works in a teaching hospital.

diabetes mellitus a complex disorder of carbohydrate, fat, and protein metabolism that is primarily a result of a deficiency or complete lack of insulin secretion by the beta cells of the pancreas or resistance to insulin (Mosby's Dictionary, p 548).

function keys special control keys on the computer keyboard.

glossary a listing of key words found in the back of some textbooks.

invoice a list showing items purchased and how much money is owed.

monitoring asking yourself if you are understanding what you are reading, watching, observing.

pulse rate the pressure on the arteries used for the counting of heartbeats.

reference a book containing information, such as an encyclopedia or a dictionary.

visualize to make a mental picture.

VOCABULARY CHECK

Directions: Choose the vocabulary word that best fits into the sentence.

1. Not knowing the meaning of the word, the student checked the _GLOSSARY_ in the back of her textbook.

2. After exercising, he put his fingers on his neck to check his _____ .

3. The student needed another _PULSE RATE_ in order to get more information for the paper she was writing.

4. She was carefully _REFERENCE_ her reading to be sure she was understanding.

5. Because he has _MONITORING_, he must be careful not to eat too much cake, cookies, and candy.

6. Along with the items she ordered from the catalogue, she found an _DIABETES MELLITUS_ in the packaging.

7. Because he knew only the _INVOICE_ answer, he did not get full credit on the test.

8. When the medical secretary remembered to use the _APPROXIMATE_ on the computer, his work went faster.
9. The _ATTENDING PHYSICIAN_ decided on the best care for the patient.
10. As she was studying for the test, she tried to _VISUALIZE_ the information on page 25 in her textbook.

WHAT IS MONITORING?

At one time or another you may have realized, after reading many pages in your textbook, that you were not really following or understanding what you had read. Although this can happen to the best readers, if it happens to you too often you may be wasting important studying time and your grades will show this.

A very good strategy for improving your reading is monitoring. When you monitor your reading, you are asking yourself if you are understanding what you are reading. In other words, you are constantly watching and observing to see if you are comprehending what you read. If the reading material is hard, you may have to ask yourself this question at the end of every sentence or paragraph. If the reading material is easier, you may need to ask yourself this question only after every section or page. The important point, however, is that as quickly as possible you become aware of when you are not understanding and then take the needed steps to improve the situation. An explanation of six comprehension-improvement strategies to help you better understand your textbooks follows.

SIX COMPREHENSION IMPROVEMENT STRATEGIES
Comprehension Improvement Strategy 1: Rereading

Many good readers have discovered that all it takes to improve their comprehension is to simply reread the passage. Usually with a second reading you are able to understand the ideas better. Sometimes it is helpful to reread the passage aloud. Listening to yourself read helps you to focus on the ideas in the selection.

EXERCISE 4–1

Directions: Read the following passage from Young and Kennedy (p. 428, underscore added). Then reread to see if you understand the instructions in the passage better. Try rereading aloud the second time and note whether or not this strategy is helpful for you.

When an item is not paid for at the time of purchase, the vendor usually includes a **packing slip** with delivery of the merchandise. A packing slip describes the items enclosed. The vendor may also enclose an invoice. An invoice describes the items and shows the amount due. Always check to verify that the items listed on the packing slip and invoice are included in the delivery.

1. Did your second reading help you understand the passage better?

   yes _____ no _____

2. Was reading the passage aloud helpful? yes _____ no _____

Comprehension Improvement Strategy 2: Learning Unknown Words

Being unfamiliar with the vocabulary or terminology in your textbooks may be the reason you are not understanding what you are reading. In some cases, you may be able to figure out the meaning or definition of the unknown word by using the surrounding words in the sentence (see Chapter 3). However, when it comes to learning a health care–related word, it will be necessary to use a dictionary or the glossary at the back of the textbook. When learning the meanings of general vocabulary words, it may be enough just to learn an approximate or nearly correct definition of the word. Then it is okay to use the surrounding words or context to supply a definition. When learning the meanings of technical words, you need to learn an exact definition. Therefore you must use some sort of reference. In either case, it will be necessary to use one of these two strategies to help you learn the meanings of unknown words in order to improve your reading comprehension.

EXERCISE 4–2

Directions: Read the following paragraph adapted from Young and Kennedy, (p. 135) and then write the meanings of any unknown words in the space provided. Show whether you used the context, dictionary, or glossary by writing "C," "D," or "G" next to the definition.

A medical assistant must understand the function of the different parts of a computer. The physical pieces that can be touched and seen are called hardware.

A monitor is a device used to display computer-generated information. A few are **monochromatic**, but most monitors today are color. The **cursor** is a pointer or flat bar appearing on the monitor that shows where the next character will appear, which is the insertion point.

For most computers, the keyboard is the primary text input device. Keyboards contain special function keys, such as the escape key, tab key, cursor movement keys, numeric keys, shift keys, and control keys.

Printers are output devices. Documents appearing on the monitor may be directed to a printer to produce a printout or **hard copy** of a document.

UNKNOWN WORD	MEANING	STRATEGY
1. _____	_____	_____
2. _____	_____	_____
3. _____	_____	_____
4. _____	_____	_____
5. _____	_____	_____

UNKNOWN WORD	MEANING	STRATEGY
6. _____	_____	_____
7. _____	_____	_____
8. _____	_____	_____
9. _____	_____	_____
10. _____	_____	_____

Comprehension Improvement Strategy 3: Making Connections

The best way to understand new information is to connect, or associate, it with facts you already know. When you are monitoring your reading and you become aware that you are not understanding, a good strategy will be to connect the topic of the selection to something you already know. Once this connection is made, you may realize that you know something about the topic already and the reading will be more understandable. The easiest way to use this strategy is to go back to the heading of the selection you do not understand and think about what it reminds you of or what you already know about the topic. See the example headings in bold print below from Young and Kennedy and note the connections that were made to each of these headings.

Example 4–1

PULSE RATE (p. 532)

Connection: **My own personal experience having my pulse rate taken by my doctor; taking my own pulse rate after I jog; pulse rate is the counting of heartbeats by feeling the pressure on the artery.**

HEART CONDUCTION (p. 898)

Connection: **The four chambers of the heart: left and right ventricles and the left and right atria, different valves that direct the flow of blood, Uncle Max's pacemaker operation.**

THE ROLE OF THE CLINICAL LABORATORY IN PATIENT CARE (p. 992)

Connection: **My old high school lab, the lab in the movie Frankenstein, microscopes, tubes, testing blood and urine, chemicals, lab coats, and complicated equipment.**

Did you notice that in these examples both facts and personal impressions were used to make the connections? When using the "making connections" strategy, associate whatever knowledge or experience you have with the topic to the heading in order to make what you are reading more understandable.

EXERCISE 4–3

Directions: Five bold-printed headings taken from Young and Kennedy are shown on p. 58. In the space provided, write you own connections to the headings. Use facts or personal experience to make the connections.

CARING FOR WOUNDS (p. 1210)

Connections: _____

_____

_____

DISINFECTION (p. 462)

Connections: _____

_____

_____

DEALING WITH SUPERVISORS (p. 1239)

Connections: _____

_____

_____

HOW FEES ARE DETERMINED (p. 258)

Connections: _____

_____

_____

THE MEDICAL ASSISTANT'S ROLE IN PEDIATRIC PROCEDURES (p. 789)

Connections: _____

_____

_____

Comprehension Improvement Strategy 4: Summarizing

When reading your textbooks, you will often see information that is technical and difficult. Sometimes the sentences will be very long and the facts will seem poorly organized and confusing. When this happens, your best strategy is to summarize the passage in your own words. To make a summary, you should briefly write down the main idea and important details from the passage (see Chapters 1 and 2). If the passage is not too long and if there is enough space, you can write the summary in the margin of your textbook. If the misunderstood passage is too long, however, it may be better to write the main ideas and important details in your notebook. When you summarize difficult ideas into your own words, you make the information easier to understand. Once the ideas are easier to understand, they will be easier to learn and you will be a more successful student.

Example 4–2

Directions: Below is an excerpt from a text by Robinson and Bird, 3rd ed (p. 194). Following that is a summary of this passage. Notice that the writer uses her own words when writing the summary. Also, she summarizes only the main idea and important details.

Infiltration anesthesia involves injecting the anesthetic solution into the tissues near the apex of the tooth to be treated. It is possible to infiltrate a maxillary tooth because the alveolus cancellous bone is porous and allows the solution to diffuse through the bone and reach the nerve at the apex of the tooth. An infiltration anesthetic can also be used to numb gingival tissues surrounding a tooth.

Infiltration anesthesia is the putting of the anesthetic solution into the tissues of the tooth that will be worked on. This method of anesthesia is good for the maxillary teeth because they are porous and the solution can easily reach the ends of the root where the nerve enters the tooth.

EXERCISE 4–4

Directions: In the space provided, summarize the following selection from Diehl, (p. 18). Remember to summarize only the main idea and important details. Use your own words and be brief.

Generally speaking, certain information is not available from the medical record for release to third parties. This information includes details of psychiatric examinations, personal history of the patient or the patient's family, and information controlled by state law. If there is a question about the content of the medical information to be released, the attending physician should be consulted regarding its accuracy or interpretation. Hospitals prefer to release information by the use of summaries or abstracts or on standard forms recommended by the American Hospital Association or local hospital groups. Duplicating an entire record is expensive; furthermore, control of the record by the hospital would be lost, and the copy might be misused. If the attending physician wishes information from the hospital record, an abstract or a copy can be given without the patient's written permission, as long as it is for the physician's own use.

_____

_____

_____

Comprehension Improvement Strategy 5: Visualizing

Another reason for not understanding what you are reading is that your mind may be wandering to other thoughts when you read your textbook. You may not be concentrating because the room you are studying in is too noisy. Or you may be thinking more about

some germs under a microscope
Rickettsia are a group of microorganisms that have some of the characteristics of
scratching dog
both bacteria and viruses. Vectors such as fleas, ticks, and mites usually transmit

pathogenic forms of rickettsia. Diseases caused by rickettsia can be treated with
deer, parks   *Western USA*
antibiotics and include Lyme disease and Rocky Mountain spotted fever, which are

both transmitted by ticks.

Figure 4–1   How a reader visualized a selection adapted from Young and Kennedy (p. 451).

the fight you had with your friend than about what you are reading, If these or similar reasons are not letting you concentrate, then using visualization as a strategy should be helpful.

When you visualize, you make a picture in your mind of what you are reading. As you read more facts from your text, you change the picture in your mind to include the new ideas. In other words, the visualizing strategy is like watching a program on the television set, only you are responsible for making the show happen by deliberately creating a picture in your mind of what you are reading. In Figure 4–1, notice the hand-written notes above the printed lines. These are examples of what one reader visualized as he read the selection.

EXERCISE 4–5

Directions: Read the following excerpt from Young and Kennedy, (p. 1019). Try to visualize the facts you are reading. Make changes to your mental picture when you read new facts. As in Figure 4-1, write what you visualize above the lines.

Normal urine color is a shade of yellow, ranging from pale straw to yellow to amber. Color

depends on the concentration of the pigment *urochrome* and the amount of water in the

specimen. A dilute specimen should be pale, and a more concentrated specimen should be a

darker yellow. Variations in color may be caused by diet, medication, and disease.

Comprehension Improvement Strategy 6: Researching

The most useful way to learn new ideas is to already have some knowledge of the subject. When you have previous knowledge of a subject, you have a base on which to build new facts. Sometimes you may not understand what you are reading because you do not know enough about the topic. If this is the case, your best strategy is to research, or learn more about the subject. One way to do this is to simply read an easier text. Or else you can check an encyclopedia or suitable health care journal in order to build up your base of knowledge. Once you have a greater general understanding about the topic you are reading, understanding your current textbook will be easier.

EXERCISE 4–6

Directions: Knowing what <u>reference</u> to read in order to learn more about your topic will make your research hunt easier. Below are two columns. On the left are different types of references you can use. These references are lettered. In the right-hand column are different topics you may read about in your textbooks. In the spaces in the right-hand column, write the letter of the reference you would use for each topic.

A. Encyclopedia

B. Easier Health Care Textbook

C. Health Care Journal

_C_ Latest information on AIDS

_B_ Health Insurance

_A_ History of Health Care

_C_ Newest Technique for Assisting with Minor Surgery

_B_ Job Training

_A_ General Nutrition

USING COMPREHENSION IMPROVEMENT STRATEGIES FOR READING YOUR TEXTBOOK

When you are actually reading your textbook and you realize that you are reading without any comprehension, you may need to use one, some, or all of the comprehension-improvement strategies discussed in this chapter. Figure 4-2 is a passage taken from Chabner, (pp. 745–746). Above the lines are handwritten notes that describe how one reader uses the different comprehension strategies to help her understand the passage better.

EXERCISE 4–7

Directions: Read the following passage taken from the textbook by Young and Kennedy, (p. 338). Using the method shown in Figure 4-2, write above the printed line the names of the comprehension strategies you used to help you understand the following paragraphs better. The comprehension strategies discussed in this chapter are

1. Rereading

2. Learning unknown words

3. Making connections

4. Summarizing

5. Visualizing

6. Researching

Workers' Compensation

All state legislatures have passed workers' compensation laws to protect wage earners against the

loss of wages and the cost of medical care resulting from occupational accident or disease. State

laws differ as to the classes of employees included and the benefits provided.

Aunt Esther's illness

Both Type 1 and Type 2 diabetes are associated with primary and secondary complications.

too much sugar, too little insulin

Primary complications of Type 1 include **ketoacidosis** and **coma** when blood sugar concen-

too little sugar

tration gets too high or the patient receives an insufficient amount of insulin. **Hypoglycemia**

occurs when too much insulin is taken by the patient. **Insulin shock** is severe hypoglycemia

caused by an overdose of insulin, decreased intake of food, or excessive exercise. Symptoms

are sweating, trembling, nervousness, irritability, and numbness. Treatment requires an

immediate dose of glucose orally or parenterally (other than through the gastrointestinal tract).

Convulsions, coma, and death can result if the diabetic person is not treated.

Secondary (long-term) **complications** appear many years after the patient develops

diabetes. These include eye disorders such as glaucoma and cataract and destruction of the

blood vessels of the retina **(diabetic retinopathy)**, causing visual loss and blindness; destruc-

tion of the kidneys **(diabetic nephropathy)**, causing renal insufficiency and often requiring

hemodialysis or renal transplantation; destruction of blood vessels, with **atherosclerosis**

leading to stroke, heart disease, and peripherovascular ischemia (gangrene, infection, and loss

of limbs); and destruction of nerves **(diabetic neuropathy)** involving pain or loss of sensation,

most commonly in the extremities. Loss of gastric motility **(gastroparesis)** also occurs.

Summary:
Two types of diabetes mellitus with two types of complications.

Primary: Ketoacidosis and coma, hypoglycemia and insulin shock.

Secondary: Destruction of the retinas, kidneys, blood vessels and
nerves, along with loss of gastric motility.

FIGURE 4–2 Example of how one reader used the various comprehension strategies in a passage adapted from Chabner ed 7 (p 745).

No state's workers' compensation laws cover all employees. However, if a patient says that he or she was injured in the workplace or is suffering from a work-associated illness, the medical assistant should check with the patient's employer to verify the insurance coverage.

Compensation benefits include medical care benefits, weekly income replacement benefits for temporary disability, permanent disability settlements, and survivor benefits when applicable. The provider of service (e.g., doctor, hospital, therapist) accepts the workers' compsensation payment as payment in full and does not bill the patient. Time limitations are set for the prompt reporting of workers' compensation cases. The employee is obligated to promptly notify the empoyer; the employer, in turn, must notify the insurance company and must refer the employee to a source of medical care.

In some states the employer and insurance company have the right to select the physician treating the patient. In essence, the purpose of workers' compensation laws is to provide prompt medical care to an injured or ill worker so that the person may be restored to health and return to full earning capacity in as short a time as possible.

REVIEWING THE LEARNING STRATEGIES

TO LEARN	USE THIS STRATEGY
Monitoring	Ask yourself if you are understanding what you are reading
To improve your reading comprehension	Rereading
	Learning unknown words
	Making connections
	Summarizing
	Visualizing
	Researching

Chapter 5

Reading the Textbook

LEARNING OBJECTIVES

In this chapter you will learn how to
- Identify and locate important features in a textbook
- Use strategies to help your concentration and comprehension when you read textbooks

VOCABULARY WORDS

The following vocabulary words are important to your understanding of the ideas in this chapter. These vocabulary words are underscored the first time they are used in the chapter. Read the list of words and definitions. Then check your understanding of these words before you read the chapter.

chaotic pertaining to being in a state of utter confusion.
credentials diplomas or certificates.
discombobulated perplexed or upset.
hypertrophy increase in volume of a tissue or organ produced entirely by enlargement of existing cells.
ingested taken in.
ions charged particles.
plaque food debris on tooth that fosters bacteria.
protein any of a large group of naturally occurring complex organic nitrogenous compounds (Mosby's Dictionary, p. 1543).
secrete to synthesize and release a substance.
statistics numerical data.

VOCABULARY CHECK

Directions: Choose the vocabulary word that best fits into the sentence.

1. The dentist tried to remove the ___PLAQUE___ from the patient's tooth.
2. She ___INGESTED___ the vitamins.
3. The glands will ___SECRETE___ a fluid.
4. ___IONS___ are charged particles associated with x-rays.
5. The tissue will ___HYPERTROPHY___ at a certain age because of hormones.
6. She had to show her ___CREDENTIALS___ before she was allowed to teach.
7. He felt all ___DISCOMBOBULATED___ when he traveled to foreign countries.
8. The student collected all the ___STATISTICS___ he could about the number of lettuces grown each year.
9. The zoo was ___CHAOTIC___ when the animals escaped from their cages.
10. It is important to get enough ___PROTEIN___ from your diet.

SURVEYING THE TEXTBOOK

Maybe you have had the experience of walking into a movie theater without knowing anything about the film being shown. Did you sit there for several minutes <u>discombobulated</u> and confused about what you were seeing on the screen? Most of the time we choose to see a movie after we have seen the previews or read reviews in magazines and newspapers. Likewise with reading your textbook. If you just start reading at Chapter 1, you may feel disconnected and bewildered about what you are reading. However, if you survey, or briefly glance through, the entire textbook before you begin your first reading assignment, you will discover that it is similar to seeing movie previews. You will know what you are getting into.

To have the time to adequately survey the text, it will be necessary to buy the book before the semester starts. Many school bookstores have their textbooks on the shelves 2 weeks or so before the semester starts. Buying your textbooks early not only will give you time to become familiar with the books but also will help you avoid the long and <u>chaotic</u> lines of students all buying their books the first day of school.

When you have your textbook, the parts that you will want to survey are

- Title page
- Table of Contents
- Bibliography
- Index
- Preface
- Glossary
- Appendix

Title Page

The title page is found at the very beginning of a book and contains some or all of the following information:

- Title
- Author—name or names and a listing of <u>credentials</u>
- Edition—if there are more than one
- Publisher
- Location or locations of the publisher's main offices

EXERCISE 5–1

Directions: Study the title page on p. 65 and then answer the following questions in the space provided.

1. The complete title of the book is <u>Clinical textbook for Vetinary tech.</u>
2. The author's name is <u>Dennis M. McCurnin</u>
3. The author has ___3___ degrees.

4. The author works at ___LSU___ University.
5. The publisher is ___Elsevier Saunders___ .
6. The coauthor is ___Joanna M. Bassert, V.MD___
7. This is the ___6th___ edition of this text.

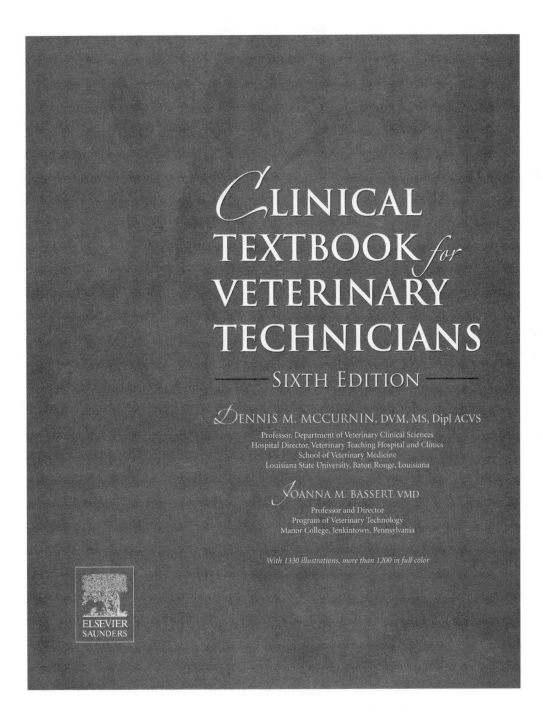

Preface

The preface ('prĕf- əs) of a textbook is found after the cover page. The preface is an introduction to the textbook and explains the author's reasons for writing the book and a description of how the book is organized. Sometimes the preface will list the names of people who helped the author write the textbook.

EXERCISE 5–2

Directions: Shown below is a preface from the Flynn textbook *Procedures in Phlebotomy*, (p. ix). Read the preface carefully and then answer the following questions.

1. For whom is this book intended? _____

2. What is the general topic for the first section? *topics directly Related to blood Collection*

3. What is the general topic for the second section? *Professional topics*

4. Where do you find the definitions of boldfaced words? *Glossary*

5. What four new additional features are included in the textbook? _____

PREFACE

As with the first and second editions, the third edition of *Procedures in Phlebotomy* is intended for students of phlebotomy. These students may be just entering the field or they may have been practicing the art of blood collection for many years. Whoever wishes to remain abreast of this rapidly changing and expanding field will find this book useful.

This edition, like the previous two, is divided into two sections, but there are many enhancements to this edition. Anatomy and Physiology (Chapter 2), has been expanded with even more relevant information for phlebotomists, as well as increased illustrative materials. Likewise, Infectious Diseases and Their Prevention (Chapter 3) contains numerous updates, including expanded phlebotomy precautions. Equipment (Chapter 4), Proper Procedures for Venipuncture (Chapter 5), and Special Collection Procedures (Chapter 6)—the crucial phlebotomy chapters— include updated information about safety equipment and many new or revised illustrations. A discussion of HIPAA is now included in Chapter 12, entitled Medical- Legal Issues and Health Law Procedures. In sum, all chapters have been reviewed, modified, and updated as warranted.

Additionally, the glossary has been expanded to define more than 150 terms; these terms once again appear in boldface throughout the text. As in the previous editions, information regarding animal phlebotomy is included as well; this subject is discussed in Appendix A. Furthermore, the review examination in Appendix C has been updated and expanded, and additional review questions have been created for many of the chapters. Throughout the book, more than 26 new and updated photographs have been added, along with many new drawings. Finally, an expanded color review chart of various blood collection tubes is included with additional information. With these enhancements and additions, I am sure students and instructors will find this text an improvement over previous editions and more useful than ever before.

Table of Contents

Surveying the table of contents is useful because it lists the topics you will be studying for the semester. The table of contents is found after the preface. It commonly contains the names of the divisions of the book: units or sections and chapters and the pages on which they start. Sometimes the chapters are divided into more specific topics that are listed as major headings. Page numbers are given for the major headings also. Because the book from which the contents on the opposite page is taken was not divided into sections or units, the contents lists only chapter titles and major headings.

Contents

x   CONTENTS

EXERCISE 5–3

Directions: Survey the table of contents from the Beaver textbook *Feline Behavior.* Then answer the following questions.

1. The book contains how many chapters? _____

2. What is the title of the fourth chapter? _____

3. On which page does the Hunting Behavior discussion begin? _____

4. In which chapter will you find a discussion of how an adult cat moves?_____

5. The Male Feline Sexual Behavior chapter contains how many major headings? _____

Glossary

The glossary is found at the end of the book and lists words and their definitions that the author believes are important. Occasionally the author will provide a key for pronouncing a word listed in the glossary.

GLOSSARY

■ ■ ■

abdomen (**ab'**-doe-men) The region of the body between the diaphragm and the pelvis.

abdominal (ab-**dom'**-ih-nal) **cavity** The superior part of the abdominopelvic cavity containing the liver, gallbladder, spleen, stomach, pancreas, small intestine, and part of the large intestine.

abdominopelvic (ab-dom'-ih-no-**pel'**-vic) **cavity** The lower part of the ventral body cavity below the thoracic cavity.

abduction (ab-**duk'**-shun) A movement whereby a body part is drawn away from the main body axis or the axis of a limb.

ABO blood types A system of categorizing blood, based on the presence or absence of specific antigens on the plasma membranes of red blood cells.

abortion (ah-**bor'**-shun) Expulsion of an embryo or fetus before it is capable of surviving outside the uterus.

absorption (ab-**sorp'**-shun) The passage of material into or through a cell or tissue, as in the movement of digested nutrients from the gastrointestinal (GI) tract into the blood or lymph.

accommodation The ability to change the curvature of the lens to clearly focus on objects at various distances.

acetylcholine (as'-eh-til-**koe'**-leen) A neurotransmitter released by cholinergic nerves, such as those stimulating skeletal muscle contraction.

Achilles' (ah-**kil'**-eez) **tendon** The tendon of the gastrocnemius and soleus muscle that inserts upon the calcaneus (heel bone).

acid (**as'**-id) A substance that is a hydrogen ion (proton) donor; dissociates in solution to produce hydrogen ions and some type of anion.

acquired immunodeficiency syndrome (AIDS) A serious disease caused by the human immunodeficiency virus (HIV) in which a deficiency develops in helper T cells.

acromegaly (ak'-roe-**meg'**-ah-lee) A condition resulting from hypersecretion of growth hormone in the adult; characterized by enlarged bones in the extremities and face along with the enlargement of other tissues.

actin (**ak'**-tin) A contractile protein found in the thin filaments within a muscle cell.

actin filaments Thin filaments composed mainly of the protein *actin;* actin and myosin filaments make up the myofibrils of muscle fibers.

action potential An electrical signal that results from depolarization of the plasma membrane in a neuron or muscle cell; also called a *nerve* or *muscle impulse.*

active immunity An acquired immunity resulting from the production of antibodies in response to exposure to antigens.

active transport The movement of substances through cell membranes against concentration gradients. Active transport requires energy expenditure.

acute (a-**kyout'**) Having a short and relatively severe course; not chronic.

Adam's apple The thyroid cartilage of the larynx. In males, it is pronounced because of enlargement caused by testosterone.

adduction (ad-**duk'**-shun) A movement whereby a body part is drawn toward the main body axis or the axis of a limb.

adenosine triphosphate (a-**den'**-oh-seen try-**fos'**-fate) **(ATP)** See *ATP.*

adipose tissue A type of connective tissue in which fat is stored.

adrenal cortex (ah-**dree'**-nal **kore'**-tekz) The outer part of the adrenal gland; it has three zones, each producing different hormones.

adrenal (ah-**dree'**-nal) **glands** Paired endocrine glands, one located just superior to each kidney. They are also known as the *suprarenal glands.*

adrenal medulla (ah-**dree'**-nal meh-**dul'**-ah) The inner part of the adrenal gland that secretes catecholamines (epinephrine and norepinephrine) in response to sympathetic stimulation.

adrenergic (ad-ren-**er'**-jik) **neuron** A neuron that releases norepinephrine.

adrenocorticotropic (ad-ree'-no-kore-ti-kow-**trope'**-ik) **hormone (ACTH)** A hormone produced by

EXERCISE 5-4

Directions: A page from the glossary of the Solomon textbook *Introduction to Human Anatomy and Physiology* (p. 293) is shown on p 69. Briefly survey the page and answer the following questions.

1. What is the first word defined in the glossary? _____

2. What is the last word defined in the glossary? _____

3. "A contractile <u>protein</u> of the thin filaments within a muscle cell" is the definition of what word? _____

4. The words in a glossary are listed in (numerical, chronological, or alphabetical) order? _____

5. "**as'**-id" is the pronunciation of what word? _____

Bibliography

The bibliography can be found at the end of each unit or chapter or at the back of the book. The bibliography lists the titles and authors of all the textbooks the writer used for writing the text. The bibliography can also be called "References."

EXERCISE 5-5

Directions: Survey the references below from the Purtilo textbook *Ethical Dimensions in the Health Professions* (p. 187). Then answer the questions that follow.

REFERENCES

1. Hippocrates. 1923. The Oath. In *Hippocrates I* (Jones, W.H.S., Trans., The Loeb Classic Library). Cambridge, MA: Harvard University Press, pp. 299–301.
2. *Griswold v Connecticut.* 1965. 381 U.S. 479. 85 S Ct. 1678.
3. Beauchamp, T.L., Childress, J. 2001. Professional-patient relationships. In *Principles of Biomedical Ethics* (5th ed.). New York: Oxford University Press, pp. 303–312.
4. Winslade, W. 2004. Confidentiality. In Post, S. (Ed.), *Encyclopedia of Bioethics* (3rd ed., vol. 4). New York: Macmillan, pp. 494–503.
5. American Medical Association. 2002. *Code of Medical Ethics.* Chicago: The Association.
6. Gutheil, T.G., Appelbaum, P.S. 1988. Confidentiality and privilege. In *Clinical Handbook of Psychiatry and the Law.* New York: McGraw-Hill, pp. 2–29.
7. Klitzman, R., Bayer, R. 2002. *Mortal Secrets. Truth and Lies in the Age of AIDS.* Baltimore: John Hopkins University Press.
8. Harman, L. 2001. *Ethical Challenges in the Management of Health Information.* Gaithersburg, MD: Aspen Publishers, Inc.
9. Sugarman, J. 2000. *20 Common Problems. Ethics in Primary Care.* New York: McGraw-Hill, pp. 158–159.
10. Randall, F., Downie, P. 1999. *Palliative Care Ethics. A Companion for all Specialties* (2nd ed.). New York: Oxford University Press, pp 152–153.
11. *Federal Register* 2002. 67:53182–53273.
12. Kulynych, J., Korn, D. 2002. The new federal medical privacy rule. *New England Journal of Medicine* 347(15):1133–1134.
13. Annas, G. 2003. HIPAA regulations—a new era of medical-record privacy? *New England Journal of Medicine* 348(15):1486–1490.

1. What is the title of the book written by Sugarman? _____

2. In what year was *Mortal Secrets. Truth and Lies in the Age of AIDS* published?

    _____

3. What edition of *Principles of Biomedical Ethics* was used?_____

4. What is the title of Harman's textbook? _____

5. The items in a bibliography are listed in (numerical, chronological, or alphabetical)

    order? _____

Appendix

The appendix that is also found in the back of the textbook contains additional information that the author did not include within the chapter. The appendix is usually ordered by letters; for example, Appendix A, Appendix B, and can contain charts, graphs, or <u>statistics</u>.

APPENDIX

B Sensory Response Development

EXERCISE 5–6

Directions: Survey Appendix B from the Beaver textbook (p. 324). List the names of the five general sensory responses illustrated in the chart.

1. _____

2. _____

3. _____

4. _____

5. _____

Index

The index is found at the very end of the textbook. It is an alphabetical listing of all the important topics in the text. The index also indicates on what page the topic can be found. For example, "cat, 561–565" means that information about cats can be found on pages 561 to 565. Another entry about cats from another textbook can look like this: "cat, 220, 223, 225." This means that information concerning cats can be found on pages 220 **and** 223 **and** 225. Indexes are particularly helpful when you are writing research papers.

EXERCISE 5–7

Directions: Look over the page from the index of the Young and Kennedy textbook *The Medical Assistant: An Applied Learning Approach* on the following page. Then answer the questions that follow.

1. The example index covers items lettered _____.

2. On what page is information about the Kling bandage found? _____

3. Into how many subtopics is "Kidney" divided? _____

4. Can names of people be included in an index? _____

5. List all the pages on which information on "Job Interview" is found. _____

_____

EXERCISE 5–8

Directions: You have now learned how to survey a textbook. Practice surveying by using this textbook or another health care textbook and answer the following questions with "yes" or "no."

1. The title page includes the edition number? _____

2. The preface discusses how many units or chapters the book is divided into? _____

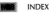 INDEX

3. The table of contents lists more than 10 chapters?_____

4. The glossary includes the pronunciation of key words?_____

5. The bibliography in the textbook is referred to as "References"?_____

6. An appendix is found at the back of the textbook?_____

7. Some topics in the index are divided into subtopics?_____

STRATEGIES FOR READING THE TEXTBOOK

Reading textbooks in the health care field requires strategies that are different from reading books for pleasure. You can learn techniques to help you to concentrate on, understand, and remember textbook information. These active reading strategies will help you to stay focused on the reading selection.

Strategies that will help you to read your textbooks with increased understanding are

- Previewing
- Questioning
- Checking health care literacy
- Reading graphic aids
- Summarizing
- Checking comprehension
- Using study guides for review

Strategies to Use Before Reading

Previewing

Before reading an assigned textbook chapter, preview the chapter. Follow these five steps:

1. Read the chapter title and ask yourself what you already know about the topic and what you want to learn about the topic.

2. Read the first paragraph and the last paragraph.

3. Read all boldface headings.

4. Pay attention to key words.

5. Look at all graphic aids such as tables, diagrams, pictures, and graphs.

These five preview steps will create a purpose for your reading. Reading with purpose will help you to concentrate as you read the chapter.

Example 5–1

Directions: Preview the following selection from Chabner's *The Language of Medicine* (p. 634). Examine the answers given for questions 1 to 3. Try to answer questions 4 and 5.

GLANDS

Sebaceous Glands

Sebaceous glands are located in the dermal layer of the skin over the entire body, with the exception of the palms (hands) and soles (feet). They secrete an oily substance called **sebum**. Sebum, containing lipids, lubricates the skin and minimizes water loss. Sebaceous glands are closely associated with hair follicles, and their ducts open into the hair follicles through which the sebum is released. Figure 16-1 shows the relationship of the sebaceous gland to the hair follicle. The sebaceous glands are influenced by sex hormones, which cause them to hypertrophy at puberty and atrophy in old age. Overproduction of sebum during puberty contributes to blackhead (comedo) formation and acne in some individuals.

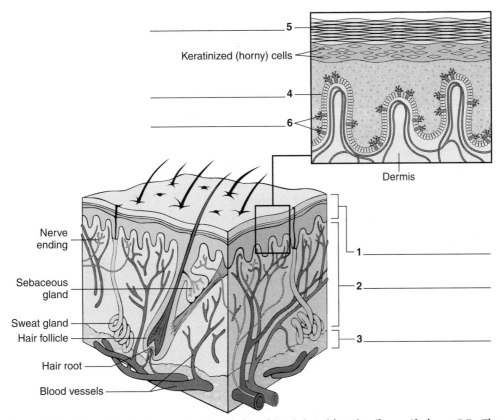

FIGURE 5-1 The skin. **(A)** Three layers of the skin. **(B)** Epidermis. (from Chabner DE: *The Language of Medicine*, ed 7, Philadelphia, Saunders, 2004, p. 631.)

Sweat Glands

Sweat glands are tiny, coiled glands found on almost all body surfaces (about 2 million in the body). They are most numerous in the palm of the hand (3000 glands per square inch) and on the sole of the foot. Figure 5-1 illustrates how the coiled sweat gland originates deep in the dermis and straightens out to extend up through the epidermis. The tiny opening on the surface is called a **pore**.

Sweat, or perspiration, is almost pure water, with dissolved materials such as salt making up less than 1 per cent of the total composition. It is colorless and odorless. The odor produced when sweat accumulates on the skin is caused by the action of bacteria on the sweat.

Sweat cools the body as it evaporates into the air. Perspiration is controlled by the sympathetic nervous system, whose nerve fibers are activated by the heart regulatory center in the hypothalamic region of the brain, which stimulates sweating.

A special variety of sweat gland, active only from puberty onward and larger than the ordinary kind, is concentrated in a few areas of the body near the reproductive organs and in the armpits. These glands (called **apocrine sweat glands**) secrete an odorless sweat, containing substances easily broken down by bacteria on the skin. The bacterial waste products produce a characteristic human body odor. The milk-producing mammary gland is another type of modified sweat gland; it secretes milk only after the birth of a child.

1. What is the topic of the reading assignment? <u>Glands</u>
2. Write the headings.

GLANDS

    <u>Sebaceous Glands</u>
    <u>Sweat Glands</u>
3. Write the definition of the key word *pore*.
    <u>The tiny opening on the surface</u>
4. Write what you already know about this topic.
    I know about sweat glands
5. Write what you will need to learn about this topic.
    What are other functions of glands?
    How do glands contribute to health?

EXERCISE 5–9

Directions: Preview the following excerpt from a health care textbook (Chabner, pp. 818 and 819). Answer the questions following the selection.

II RADIOLOGY
A. Characteristics of X-Rays

Several characteristics of x-rays are useful to physicians in the diagnosis and treatment of disease. Some of these characteristics are the following:

1. **Ability to cause exposure of a photographic plate.** If a photographic plate is placed in front of a beam of x-rays, the x-rays, traveling unimpeded through the air, will expose the silver coating of the plate and cause it to blacken.
2. **Ability to penetrate different substances to varying degrees.** X-rays pass through the different types of substances in the human body (air in the lungs, water in blood vessels and lymph, fat around muscles, and metal such as calcium in bones) with varying ease. Air is the least dense substance and exhibits the greatest transmission. Fat is dense, water is next, followed by metal, which is the densest and transmits least. If the x-rays are absorbed (stopped) by the denser body substance (e.g., calcium in bones), they do not reach the photographic plate held behind the patient, and white areas are left in the x-ray film (plate). Figure 5-2 is an example of an x-ray photograph.

    A substance is said to be **radiolucent** if it permits passage of most of the x-rays. Lung tissue (containg air) is an example of a radiolucent substance, and it appears black on an x-ray image. **Radiopaque** substances (bones) are those that absorb most of the x-rays they are exposed to, allowing only a small fraction of the x-rays to reach the x-ray plate. Thus, normally radiopaque, calcium-containing bone appears white on an x-ray image.
3. **Invisibility.** X-rays cannot be detected by sight, sound, or touch. Workers exposed to x-rays must wear a **film badge** to detect and record the amount of radiation to which they have been exposed. The film badge contains a special film that is exposed by x-rays. The amount of blackness on the film is an indication of the amount of x-rays or gamma rays received by the wearer.
4. **Travel in straight lines.** This property allows the formation of precise shadow images on the x-ray plate and also permits x-ray beams to be directed accurately at a tissue site during radiotherapy.

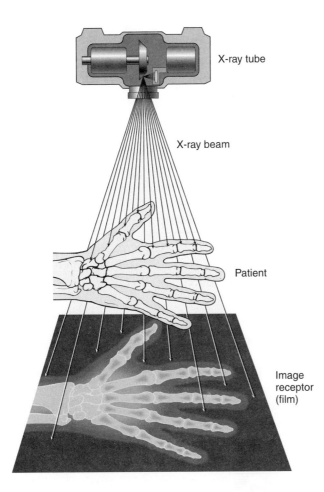

X-ray tube

X-ray beam

Patient

Image receptor (film)

FIGURE 5-2 X-ray photograph (radiograph) of the hand. Relative position of x-ray to be, patient (hand), and film necessary to make the x-ray photograph is shown. Bones tend to stop diagnostic x-rays, but soft tissue does not. This results in the light and dark regions that form the image. (from Chabner DE: *The Language of Medicine*, ed. 7, Philadelphia, Saunders, 2004, p 819.)

5. **Scattering of radiation**. Scattering occurs when x-rays come in contact with any material. Greater scatter occurs with dense objects and less scatter with those substances that are radiolucent. In addition, because scatter can blur images and expose areas of film that otherwise would be in shadow, a grid (containing thin lead strips arranged parallel to the x-ray beams) is placed in front of the film to absorb scattered radiation before it strikes the x-ray film.

6. **Ionization**. X-rays have the ability to ionize substances through which they pass. Ionization is a chemical process in which the energy of an x-ray beam causes rearrangement and disruption within a substance, so that previously neutral particles are changed to charged particles called **ions**. This strongly ionizing ability of x-rays is a double-edged sword. In x-ray therapy, the ionizing effect of x-rays can help kill cancerous cells and stop tumor growth; however, ionizing x-rays in small doses can affect normal body cells, leading to tissue damage and malignant changes. Thus, persons exposed to high doses of x-ray are at risk of developing leukemia, thyroid tumors, breast cancer, or other malignancies.

1. What is the topic of the reading assignment? _____

2. How many characteristics are listed? _____

3. Write the definition of the key word ions. _____

_____

4. Write what you already know about this topic. _____

5. Write what you need to learn about this topic. _____

_____

_____

Questioning

Try to think about the main ideas that will be covered in the assignment. Ask questions to help you identify these main ideas as you read. Asking questions helps you to read with a purpose. Your goal while reading is to answer your questions. Asking questions will help you to

- Identify the concepts and facts that you still need to learn.
- Think about and evaluate the information you are reading.
- Remember important details.

A good method is to turn to boldface headings into questions

Example 5–2

Directions: Look at the following example of formulating questions from a boldface heading.

Diseases of Red Blood Cells

1. What are the diseases of red blood cells?
2. How are the diseases of red blood cells treated?

Looking for answers to your questions will help you concentrate as you read text-books.

EXERCISE 5–10

Directions: Read the following heading.

Patient Registration System

Write two questions that you could ask about this heading.

1. _____

2. _____

Strategies to Use While Reading

Asking the 5W Questions

You can use the following 5W questions to help you focus on your textbook assignments. The 5Ws will help you to identify the main ideas and important details as you read. These 5W questions will help you to understand the most important information in the selection. You will not be discouraged by complicated sentence structure and difficult vocabulary if you use the 5W questions to give you the essential information in your reading assignments.

1. Who or what is the assigned reading about? (The answer to this question helps you to identify the topic, or subject, of the reading assignment.)
2. What is the main point being made about the subject? (The answer to this question is the main idea.)
3. When? (The answer to this question helps you to locate the important details.)
4. Where? (The answer to this question helps you to locate the important details.)
5. Why? or How? (The answer to this question helps you to locate the important details.)

At times, not all of the details are given in a selection. Therefore, you may not always find the answers to all of the 5Ws. Use the 5W questions to keep you actively involved as you read.

Read each chapter section by section. Stop at the end of each section to check your comprehension by trying to answer the 5W questions. You might want to write these answers or other notes in the margin of your textbook. Note taking helps you to become an active reader.

Example 5–3

Directions: Read the following excerpt from the Young and Kennedy health care textbook *The Medical Assistant An Applied Approach* (p. 58). Review the 5W questions and the answers to these questions.

TIME MANAGEMENT

We have often heard the expression "work smart." This means that we are to use our time efficiently and concentrate on the duties that are most important first. To do this we must first prioritize our duties and arrange our schedule to ensure that these duties can be performed (see the next section). The first way to improve time management is to plan the tasks that need to be done that day. Taking 10 minutes to write down the day's tasks will help to ensure that they are done. Then it is important to stay on schedule throughout the day, unless emergencies disrupt the schedule. Even then, when office days are well planned, allowances can be made for emergencies, even if they happen often, and the majority of the tasks can still be completed. The key to managing time is prioritizing.

1. Who or what? *Time Management*
2. What is the main point being made about the subject? *To use time efficiently, duties must be prioritized*
3. When? *Every day*
4. Where? *At the office*
5. Why? *To concentrate on duties that are most important first*

EXERCISE 5–11

Directions: Read the following selection from Chabner's textbook (p. 772) and answer the 5W questions.

DNA has two main functions in a normal cell. First, DNA controls the production of new cells (cell division). When a cell divides, the DNA material in each chromosome copies itself so that exactly the same DNA is passed to the two new daughter cells that are formed. This process of cell division is called **mitosis**.

Second, between cycles of mitosis, DNA controls the production of new proteins (**protein synthesis**) in the cell.

1. Who or what is the assigned reading about? _____

2. What is the main point being made about the subject? _____

   _____

3. When? _____

4. Where? _____

5. Why or how? _____

Assessing Your Health Care Literacy

Be aware of your literacy level in the health care fields. To be literate in the health care field, you have to have the ability to read the textbooks and write about the information you are learning. You should also be able to apply this information to job related tasks in the health fields.

You may have difficulty with the vocabulary in your textbooks because there are many technical terms to learn. Vocabulary meanings in the health care fields have to be precise. You have to learn technical terms and abbreviations and symbols for these terms to understand the reading material. You cannot simply skip over difficult vocabulary. You should learn new technical words as you come to them when you read your textbooks. When you come across a new technical word in your health care textbooks, apply these strategies:

1. Try to see if the word is defined in context.
2. If you cannot determine the meaning from context clues, use the glossary or index of your textbook.
3. If you cannot find the word meaning within the textbook, use the dictionary of allied health terms or a technical dictionary.
4. When you have found the meanings of the new words, reread the assignment. You will now have a much better understanding of the chapter.

Example 5–4

Read the following excerpt from a health care textbook (Chabner, p. 37). Reread the excerpt after you have learned the meanings of the words in boldface.

Differences in Cells. Cells are different, or specialized, throughout the body to carry out their individual functions. For example, a **muscle cell** is long and slender and contains fibers that aid in contracting and relaxing; an **epithelial cell** (a lining and skin cell) may be square and flat to provide protection; a **nerve cell** may be long and have various fibrous extensions that aid in its job of carrying impulses; a **fat cell** contains large empty spaces for fat storage. These are only a few of the many types of cells in the body.

1. *Muscle* cell: long and slender and contains fibers that aid in contracting and relaxing
2. *Epithelial* cell: A lining and skin cell, may be square and flat to provide protection

3. *Nerve* cell: may be quite long and have numerous fibrous extensions that aid in its job of carrying impulses

4. *Fat* cell: contains large empty spaces for fat storage

Learning the meanings of these terms helps you to understand the main idea of the selection, which is that different cells are specialized to carry out their specific functions.

EXERCISE 5–12

Directions: Read the following excerpt from the Chabner health care textbook (p. 444). Write the meaning of each word in boldface. Reread the excerpt after you have learned the word meanings. Then write the main idea of the selection.

The lungs extend from the collarbone to the **diaphragm** in the thoracic cavity. The diaphragm is a muscular partition separating the thoracic from the abdominal cavity and aiding in the process of breathing. It contracts and descends with each **inhalation (inspiration)**. The downward movement of the diaphragm enlarges the area in the thoracic cavity, decreasing internal air pressure, so that air flows into the lungs to equalize the pressure. When the lungs are full, the diaphragm relaxes and elevates, making the area in the thoracic cavity smaller, thus increasing the air pressure in the chest. Air then is expelled out of the lungs to equalize the pressure; this is called **exhalation (expiration)**. Figure 5-3 shows the position of the diaphragm in inspiration and expiration.

WORD   **MEANING**

1. Diaphragm   _____

2. Inhalation   _____

3. Exhalation   _____

MAIN IDEA

4. _____

Reading Graphic Aids

Health care textbooks are filled with graphic aids: pictures, graphs, tables, and diagrams. You should carefully read this material so that you can succeed in your studies.

Graphic materials are designed to be clear so you can use these aids to help you concentrate on and learn new information. The following five strategies allow you to use graphic aids to help you better understand and read your textbooks.

1. Read the title carefully to determine the subject of the graphic aid.

2. Check the vocabulary. Learn the meaning of each word in the headings, labels, and captions so that you will understand the information.

3. Figure out the purpose of the graphic aid. Think about how it relates to the ideas discussed in the chapter. Work back and forth between the picture and the

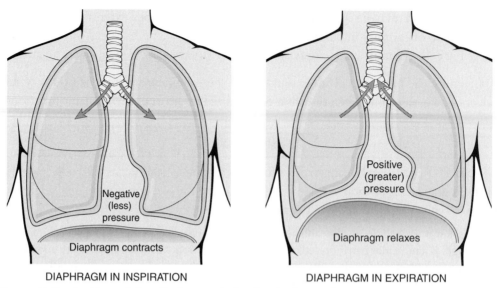

FIGURE 5-3 Position of the diaphragm during inspiration and expiration. During inspiration air flows in as the chest cavity enlarges. During expiration air flows out as the chest cavity becomes smaller. (From Chabner DE: *The Language of Medicine*, ed 7, Philadelphia, Saunders, 2004 p 445.)

written text. Determining the relationship between the two will help you to understand the information you need to learn.

4. If the graphic aid has a number or symbol, think about what each item represents.
5. Paraphrase the ideas in the picture into language you understand.

Read graphic aids carefully to help you concentrate on, understand, and remember textbook information.

Example 5–5

Read and study Figure 5-3, a graphic aid from Chabner (p. 445), and the answers that are provided to the questions.

1. What is the subject of the diagram? *Comparison of the diaphragm in inspiration and expiration.*
2. What symbols are being used to illustrate the comparison? *Arrows*
3. Define inspiration. *Breathing in*
4. Define expiration. *Breathing out*
5. When air flows out, is the chest cavity larger or smaller? *Smaller*

EXERCISE 5–13

Directions: Read and study Table 5-1, a graphic aid from the Robinson and Bird textbook *Essentials of Dental Assisting* (p. 280). Answer the questions and write your answers in the space provided.

1. What is the title of this table? _____
2. What vitamins are listed in this table? _____

TABLE 5–1 Fat-Soluble Vitamins

Vitamin	Important Functions	Best Sources	Deficiency Symptoms
Vitamin A	Growth Health of the eyes Structure and functioning of the cells of the skin and mucous membranes Promotes health of the oral structures	Fish liver oils Liver Green and yellow vegetables Fruit (yellow) Butter, milk, cream, cheese Egg yolk	Retarded growth Night blindness Increased susceptibility to infections Changes in skin and mucous membranes
Vitamin D	Helps absorb calcium from digestive tract and build calcium and phosphorus into bones and teeth Growth	Vitamin D–irradiated milk Fish liver oil Sunshine on skin	Rickets Poor tooth development
Vitamin E	Protects vitamin A and essential fatty acids from oxidation Aids in the formation of red blood cells, muscles, and other tissues	Wheat germ oil Vegetable oils Green vegetables Milk fat, butter Egg yolk	Undetermined
Vitamin K	Normal clotting of blood Helps maintain normal liver function	Green leafy vegetables Liver Soybean and other vegetable oils Synthesized by intestinal bacteria	Hemorrhages

From Bird D, Robinson D: Torres and Ehrlich Modern Dental Assisting, ed 6, Philadelphia, Saunders, 1999.

3. Hemorrhages are a deficiency symptom of vitamin _____

4. What information is summarized in this table? _____

   _____

5. Look for two vocabulary words in Table 5-1 that you need to learn. Write the words, their definitions, and your source for finding the word meanings.

WORD	DEFINITION	SOURCE
1._____	_____	_____
2. _____	_____	_____

Summarizing

Check your comprehension by answering the 5W questions. Your answers will give you a summary of each topic. Paraphrase the ideas of the text into language you understand. Make sure that you understand each topic before you go on to the next boldface heading.

Strategies for Reading Difficult Passages

Sometimes, the textbook assignment may seem difficult and you are tempted to give up. Take a short break and then try these strategies to help you interpret complicated reading.

1. Read carefully. Do not skip any information.
2. Work methodically. Much of the information is presented step by step. Follow the order of the selection so that you are not confused.
3. Go over the vocabulary. Make sure that you have learned all the new words.
4. Ask questions. Formulating questions can help you to clarify your thinking.
5. Reread the section, looking for the main idea and the most important details.

Strategies to Use After Reading

When you have finished reading the chapter one topic at a time, look at the assignment as a whole.

- Underline the main idea and the important details that you want to remember.
- Write a summary, outline, or map of the main ideas and important details that you can use to review the chapter. This written summary or outline will serve as a study guide.
- Study the important ideas of the chapter. Review underlined text material, summaries, outlines, maps, and notes.
- Answer the review questions at the end of each chapter. Correct your answers.
- Design your own test based on the reading assignments.

Answer the questions on this practice test and correct your answers. Taking practice tests will help you to remember the information so that you will improve your test grades.

EXERCISE 5–14

Directions: Use all the reading strategies you learned in this chapter to concentrate on, understand, and remember textbook information. The questions and directions in this exercise will help you guide your reading of the following selection from a health care textbook (Robinson and Bird, p. 283-284).

PREVENTIVE DENTAL CARE
Patient Education

Patient education in oral health is the responsibility of all members of the dental health care team. It occurs at every appointment beginning with the initial examination and continues with every visit. An oral health education program is based upon **motivation** and **education**.

Motivation

The dental health professional should work with the patient to increase his or her motivational level so the patient *wants* to learn and is *willing* to do the things necessary to achieve and maintain oral health. The lower the patient's level of motivation, the less the chance of success for his or her oral hygiene program.

The first step is to help the patient recognize that he or she has a problem that needs to be solved. Then it is necessary for the patient to accept his or her role in solving the problem. As an example, the patient may not know that improper toothbrushing can damage the teeth and gums. Once the patient recognizes the problem and is willing to change his or her behavior, he or she will be more motivated to learn how to use the proper techniques.

Education

Oral health education is not a lecture. It is listening more than talking, and involves more problem solving than instruction. It is creating in the patient an awareness of the need to return regularly for professional prophylaxis, examination, and treatment.

It is helping parents recognize the importance of preventive steps, such as the placement of sealants and the use of fluorides.

It is counseling to increase the patient's awareness of the role of nutrition in achieving optimum dental and general health.

In your role as a dental health educator, you must be enthusiastic about helping others achieve optimum oral health.

Acceptance. The patient can learn more easily when he or she feels safe, accepted, and respected. Encouragement is given freely, and correction is structured in a positve manner. Most important, the patient is *never* scolded, embarrassed or teased because of his or her ignorance or errors.

Active Learning. The most productive form of learning occurs when the patient is actively participating in the process, utilizing as many of his or her senses as possible. Teaching plaque control is an ideal situation for **active learning**.

TABLE 5–2   Hard Facts About Soft Drinks

1. Large sizes mean more calories, more sugar, and more acid in a single serving. A 64-ounce "big cup" has more than five 12-ounce cans in a single serving.
2. Soft drinks have no nutritional value. In regular sodas, all the calories come from sugar.
3. Sugar in sodas combines with bacteria in the mouth to form acid.
4. Diet or "sugar-free" sodas contain their own acid. The acid attacks the teeth. Each acid attack lasts about 20 minutes.
5. In addition to tooth decay, heavy soda consumption has been linked to diabetes, obesity, and osteoporosis.
6. Teenagers today drink three times more soda than teenagers 20 years ago, often as a substitute for milk.
7. One fifth of all 1- and 2-year old children drink sodas.
8. Sealants protect only the chewing surfaces of teeth. Decay caused by sodas tends to occur on smooth tooth surfaces, where sealants cannot reach.

Modified from the Minnesota Dental Association.

I. Before Reading
   A. Previewing
      1. Read the heading and subheadings to identify the topic. Write the topic in the space provided. _____
      2. Read the first and last paragraphs.
      3. Write the meaning of these key words.
         a. Motivation_____
         b. Education _____
      4. What fraction of 1- and 2- year olds drink soda? _____
      5. Think about what you already know about this topic. Write what you still need to know. _____
         _____
         _____

   B. Questioning
      6. Based on your preview, formulate questions from the heading of the reading selection. _____
         _____

II. While reading
      7. Ask the 5W questions. Read the selection with the goal of answering your question. Stop at each boldface heading to check your comprehension.
      8. Think about the order of the information. Which did you learn about first, how to motivate or educate your patients? _____
      9. What is the subject of the table? _____
      10. How does this table relate to the written text? _____
   A. Summarizing
      11. Answer your 5W questions. Remember to check your comprehension as you complete each topic. Paraphrase the author's information in your own words to reinforce your understanding of the information. _____
         _____
         _____
         _____
         _____

III. After Reading
   A. Underline
      12. **Underline** the main ideas and important details that you will want to remember.
   B. Write
      13. **Write** a summary or outline or map the main ideas and important details of the selection.

C. Study

14. **Review** your underlined material and study guides. Design a practice test. Correct your answers.

REVIEWING READING THE TEXTBOOK

TO LEARN	USE THIS STRATEGY
How to identify and locate important information in your textbook	Survey the following features: 1. Title page 2. Preface 3. Table of contents 4. Glossary 5. Bibliography 6. Appendix 7. Index
Previewing	1. Read the title 2. Read the first and last paragraphs 3. Read all boldface headings 4. Pay attention to key words 5. Look at all graphic aids
Questioning	Turn boldface headings into questions
To concentrate while reading	Ask 5W questions
To check health care literacy	Learn technical vocabulary words
To read graphic aids	1. Read the title 2. Check the vocabulary 3. Figure out the purpose of the graphic aid 4. Learn what the numbers or symbols represent 5. Paraphrase the ideas into your own words
To summarize	Answer the 5W questions
How to understand difficult passages	1. Do not skip information 2. Follow the order of the information 3. Learn all new vocabulary words 4. Ask questions 5. Reread the selection
To review the chapter as a whole	Underline, write summary, or map main ideas and important details. Review study guides. Take practice tests.

UNIT II

WRITING STRATEGIES

Many students feel that they need to improve their writing skills. Most students can improve their writing with practice and by learning that writing is a process. Unit II, Writing Strategies, guides students through the steps of the writing process. Chapter 6, Organizing Ideas, will teach you how to use prewriting strategies to develop a plan for writing. Chapter 7, Writing the First Draft, will demonstrate how you put all your ideas on paper by following your writing plan. Chapter 8, Revising the Final Draft, will guide you through the steps of revision, editing, and proofreading. You will also be reminded of some problem areas to avoid in spelling, grammar, capitalization, and punctuation. Following the steps in the writing process will help you to develop an improved final paper.

Chapter 6

Organizing Ideas

LEARNING OBJECTIVES

In this chapter you learn how to
- Use prewriting strategies
- Develop a plan for writing

VOCABULARY WORDS

The following vocabulary words are important to your understanding of the ideas in this chapter. These vocabulary words are <u>underscored</u> the first time they are used in the chapter. Read the list of words and definitions. Then check your understanding of these words before you read the chapter.

abuse harmful treatment.
audience the people who will read your writing.
brainstorming spontaneously formulating ideas.

E-mail or electronic mail a message sent on a computer.
form the medium for the written message.
narrating telling a story.
prewriting plan for writing.
process the several steps involved in doing something.
purpose why the author is writing.
subject the topic.

VOCABULARY CHECK

Directions: Choose the vocabulary word that best fits into the sentence.

1. Tony learned to use _____ strategies to develop a writing plan.

2. You cannot do everything at once; each step is part of a total _____.

3. Mrs. Jonas decided to use the _____ of a manual when she wrote the directions for the use of the new computer program.

4. Have you established your _____ for writing this outline?

5. As the storyteller was _____ the tale, everyone listened intently.

6. Thelma received your message on _____ before she received the letter.

7. The topic, or _____, of your report is a crucial issue today.

8. The _____ listened to the speaker's report and then criticized the information.

9. Veronica finds _____ helpful as she collects information about her topic.

10. Verbal _____ can be damaging to a child's self esteem.

THE WRITING PROCESS

Many students find it difficult to start a writing assignment. They are overwhelmed by the task of writing because they try to do the planning, drafting, revising, editing, and proofreading in just one step.

Writing is a <u>process</u> of many steps. These steps include the following:

- **Step 1: Prewriting**
  You select a subject, collect details about the subject, and develop your writing plan.
- **Step 2: Writing the First Draft**
  You organize your ideas into sentences and paragraphs.
- **Step 3: Revising**
  You make the changes necessary to improve your writing.
- **Step 4: Editing and Proofreading**
  You examine your writing for any specific errors in spelling, punctuation, grammar, or style. Check your paper carefully and correct any errors before you hand in your final draft.

If you learn the strategies involved in each of these steps in the writing process, you will be more successful in completing your writing assignments.

PREWRITING STRATEGIES

<u>Prewriting</u> strategies help you to develop a plan for writing. This plan will be your guide when you are ready to write your first draft. Your writing plan should include the following:

1. The <u>Subject</u>: The subject answers the question **who?** or **what?** The subject is the topic you will write about.
2. The <u>Purpose</u>: The purpose answers the question **why?** Why are you writing? Are you writing to **explain, to describe, to persuade,** or to **narrate?**
3. <u>Form</u>: Form answers the question **what?** What are you writing? Form is the medium through which you express your ideas.
4. <u>Audience</u>: The people who read your writing make up the audience. Think about your readers. You should always direct your information to a specific audience for clear, direct writing.

If you begin all your writing assignments by following this plan, you will be getting off to a good start.

Example 6–1

One student's writing plan:

Subject: Child <u>abuse</u>
Purpose: To persuade your readers of the danger of child abuse
Form: Report
Audience: Nursing Assistants

EXERCISE 6–1

Directions: Develop your own writing plan. Fill in the following information:

Subject: _____

Purpose: _____

Form: _____

Audience: _____

SELECTING A SUBJECT

Think about who or what you want to write about. Then list words or ideas that relate to your subject. This step is called <u>brainstorming</u>. It means that you are thinking of everything you know about your chosen subject so that you can collect information about this topic.

COLLECTING DETAILS

An effective strategy for collecting details about your subject is to ask and answer the 5W questions.

Example 6–2

Ask and answer the 5W questions:

1. **Who or what?** Child abuse.
2. **What is the main point being made about the subject?** Child abuse is a major cause of child injury and death.
3. **When?** Currently on the increase.
4. **Where?** The United States.
5. **Why or how?** Abusive parents and failure of health professionals to report previous, less serious injuries.

EXERCISE 6–2

Directions: Collect details about your subject by asking and answering the 5W questions.

Who or what? _____

What is the main point being made about the subject? _____

_____

When?_____

Where? _____

Why or how? _____

ORGANIZING YOUR INFORMATION

Once you have answered the 5W questions, you are ready to organize your information. You can organize the details around your subject by

• **Mapping**   • **Listing**   • **Writing a topic outline**

Example 6–3

Different ways a student could organize details around a subject:

1. **Mapping:** Map your ideas. Begin to map your ideas with your subject in the middle. Add the details that relate to your subject.

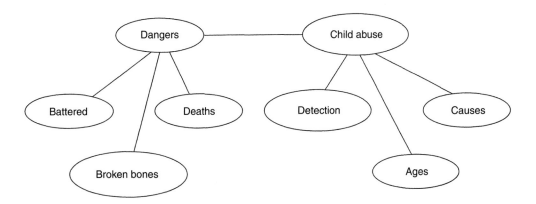

2. **Listing:** Child abuse is a major cause of injury and death to children.

   - Burns
   - Bruises
   - Broken bones
   - Sexual abuse
   - Death
   - Prevention

3. **Writing a topic outline:** Dangers to children caused by child abuse.

   a. Major physical injuries
      (1) Burns
      (2) Bruises
      (3) Broken bones
   b. Lasting emotional trauma
      (1) Sexual abuse
      (2) Emotional abuse
   c. High death rates
   d. How to prevent abuse
      (1) Early detection
      (2) Immediate reporting

EXERCISE 6–3

Directions: Review your collection of details that you gathered by asking and answering the 5W questions. Decide which method of organizing details around your subject will work the best for you. Organize your details by mapping, listing, or writing a topic outline.

PLANNING THE MAIN IDEA

Enlarge your subject into a main idea by answering the first 2 of the 5W questions:

- **Who** or **what** are you writing about? = **Subject**
- **What** do you want to say about the subject? = **Main Idea**

Example 6–4

- **Who** or **what**? = Child abuse
- **What** is being said about child abuse? = Child abuse is a major cause of children's injury and death in the United States.

EXERCISE 6–4

Directions: Fill in the following information so that you can formulate the main idea of your writing:

- **Who or what?** _____
- **What** are you saying about the subject? _____

_____

DECIDING ON YOUR PURPOSE

Why are you writing? Your purpose should be related to your main idea. For example, if a writer wants to convey to readers that child abuse is a major cause of children's injury and death, the purpose would be to **persuade** the readers of all the dangers of child abuse. The facts collected would be included to sway the reader toward the writer's point of view. The facts and examples that are given are collected to persuade your readers to agree with your opinion.

Example 6–5

The details collected are to **persuade** the reader that child abuse is dangerous.

EXERCISE 6–5

Directions: Choose your purpose. Why are you writing? Fill in your map, list, or outline so that the details you collect will reflect your purpose.

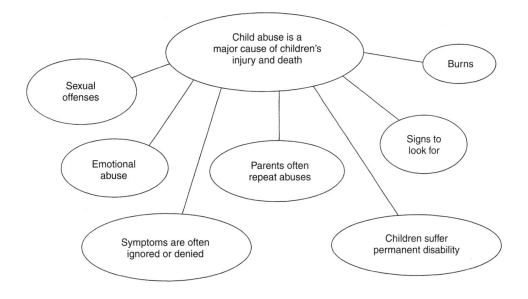

ORGANIZING INFORMATION ACCORDING TO PURPOSE

Your organization should be related to your purpose in writing. Choose a plan of organization that will fulfill your purpose. Some types of organization plans are:

- **Describing:** You give many details. You might be describing people, places, or objects.
- **Explaining:** You are explaining "how to" or "giving causes" or "definitions." When you are explaining, the facts you choose give information about the object or process you are writing about.
- **Persuading:** You are persuading when you are trying to convince someone that he or she should agree with your opinion. You might be persuading when you are writing about reasons for following procedures or for changing existing conditions. When you are persuading, you collect details to back up your opinion.
- Narrating: You are narrating when you are giving details about an experience you want to share. You might narrate an encounter with a patient or an employer. When you are narrating, sequence is important.

CHOOSING THE FORM

Once you have chosen your main idea, purpose, and organization plan, think about the most effective form to use to communicate your ideas. Look over Table 6–1 and choose the form that would best convey your message.

TABLE 6–1   Some Sample Forms for Writing

Descriptions	Requests
Directions	Case studies
Letters	E-mail
Memos	Lab reports
Pamphlets	Observation reports
Brochures	Patient histories or profiles
Captions for pictures	Summaries
Charts	Add other forms _____
Proposals	_____
Reports	

EXERCISE 6–6

Directions: Choose the form that would communicate your main idea most effectively.

_____

Write why you have chosen this form _____

CHOOSING THE AUDIENCE

Who will read your writing? Will your reader be your instructor, your employer, a coworker, a classmate, or yourself? Your writing will be improved if you direct your message toward a specific audience. Think about your audience when you are organizing your information.

EXERCISE 6–7

Directions: List your audience. Why did you choose this audience? _____

_____

_____

Now it is your turn to be the audience. When you read the following selections, try to uncover the writer's plan. You can then try to model your writing around those plans that you can identify.

Example 6–7

Read the following selection from *EMT Prehospital Care* by Henry and Stapleton (p. 241) and the answers given for the writer's plan.

PULSE CHECK

After checking responsiveness, airway, and breathing, you should check the patient for a pulse. Check the carotid pulse on any patient who is unresponsive. For responsive patients, the radial pulse is assessed for rate and quality. If it is faint or absent, check the carotid pulse. If the patient is younger than 1 year of age, palpate a brachial pulse. You should check for a femoral pulse if the brachial pulse is faint or absent.

Subject: *Pulse check.*
Main Idea: *Different pulses are checked for different reasons.*
Purpose: *Describing.*
Form: *Description*
Audience: *You.*

EXERCISE 6–8

Directions: Read the following selections and fill in the blanks to identify the writer's plan.

CASE IN POINT

A patient with a head wound has had a dressing applied on the skull above the ear with a pressure bandage wrapped around the head. The bandage and dressing were soaked with blood. On arrival at the hospital, the patient stated, "I am going to pass out" —an ominous statement in a patient with blood loss. His blood pressure was 60 by palpation. The dressing was removed and revealed spurting blood from the temporal artery, which was quickly and completely controlled with *focused direct pressure*. After subsequent repair of the wound and restoration of blood volume, the patient made a full recovery from what otherwise might have become a fatal scalp wound (Henry and Stapleton, pp. 546-547).

Subject: _____

Main Idea: _____

_____

Purpose: _____

Form: _____

Audience: _____

PRINTER PAPER

The chart is a record of care rendered and the patient's response to care during hospitalization. The nursing unit to which the patient is assigned adds forms to the chart. The record is a legal document and should be maintained as such. Standard forms are placed on all patients' charts; supplemental forms may be added according to the need dictated by each patient's treatment and care. The purpose of the forms is the same for each hospital, but the sequence of forms in the chart and the placement of blank forms that are added may differ from hospital to hospital.

The information contained in the patient's chart must always be regarded as confidential. (LeFleur Brooks and Gillingham, p. 155).

Subject: _____

Main Idea: _____

_____

Purpose: _____

Form: _____

Audience: _____

CARDIAC ARREST

Cardiac arrest occurs when the patient's heart goes into a rhythm that does not generate blood flow. This may include **asystole** (flatline), where there is no electrical activity or contraction of the heart; **pulseless electrical activity,** where there is an organized electrical heart rhythm but no palpable pulse; or ventricular fibrillation. Ventricular fibrillation is the most common cause of sudden cardiac arrest in adults. Because time to defibrillation is the most critical treatment variable for survival from ventricular fibrillation, activation of the emergency medical services (EMS) system and application of an AED are the most important actions taken for the victim of cardiac arrest. The EMT is trained to recognize the need for AED use to increase the patient's chance of survival (Henry and Stapleton, pp. 382-383).

Subject: _____

Main Idea: _____

_____

Purpose: _____

Form: _____

Audience: _____

REVIEWING ORGANIZING IDEAS

TO LEARN	USE THIS STRATEGY
To develop a plan for writing	Use prewriting strategies
To select a subject	Ask yourself who or what you want to write about
To collect details about the subject	Ask the 5W questions
To organize the details	Map, list, or outline your information
To plan the main idea	Ask yourself what you want to say about the subject
To decide on the purpose	Ask yourself why you are writing
To choose an organization plan	Decide whether you want to describe, explain, persuade, or narrate
To select the form	Choose the medium for your writing

TO LEARN

To choose the audience

To construct a writing plan

USE THIS STRATEGY

Decide who will read your writing.
Direct your writing toward those readers

Outline your
Subject
Main Idea
Purpose
Form
Audience

Chapter
7

Writing the First Draft

LEARNING OBJECTIVES

In this chapter you will learn how to
• Write the first draft

VOCABULARY WORDS

These vocabulary words are important to your understanding the ideas in this chapter. These vocabulary words are <u>underscored</u> the first time they are used in the chapter. Read the list of words and definitions. Then check your understanding of these words before you read the chapter.

confidence self-assurance.
detect to see.
draft a rough version of written work.
emphasis stresses the importance of something.
endangered subject to being destroyed.

expanded expressed in greater detail.
product the end result of the creative effort of writing.
revision rewriting.
sequence the order of events.
slanted biased.

VOCABULARY CHECK

Directions: Choose the vocabulary word that best fits into the sentence.

1. This work is the _____ of many years effort.

2. My first _____ needed to be changed.

3. Diane has the _____ as well as the ability needed to accept the leading role in the play.

4. Margaret's _____ of her first paper was well organized.

5. Barry _____ his ideas so that we could understand his message.

6. Environmentalists want to protect _____ species.

7. That article is _____ towards the writer's point of view.

8. The _____ of the story is easy to follow.

9. It's easy for Raymond to _____ the problem, but does he know how to solve it?

10. The _____ on the cost of health care outweighs other issues.

INTRODUCTION

Writing the first <u>draft</u> is when you, the writer, put all your ideas on paper. Remember, your first draft is not your finished <u>product</u>. Once you learn that writing is a process and that your first draft is not the end product, you will not have to worry about making the first draft perfect. This realization should take away your feelings of anxiety when you have a writing assignment. Remember that the writing process breaks the task of writing into manageable steps.

GETTING STARTED

Sometimes, students find it difficult to get started on the first draft. Begin your first draft while all the ideas are fresh in your mind and you can get all these thoughts on paper. Start your first draft when you have realistically set up enough time to finish. It's best to work on your first draft uninterrupted. Don't attempt to initiate this step of the writing process if you know that in five or ten minutes you'll have to leave for a class or your job. Don't stop your work to answer phone calls or watch television. Find a place to work where you can write freely, away from distractions and interruptions. Realizing that you are not expected to write a perfect first draft should give you the <u>confidence</u> to get started.

Look over your writing plan. You've selected your **subject, purpose, form** and **audience.** Expand this plan by developing your main ideas into sentences and paragraphs. Write freely. Remember, you'll have time to make your changes in the next step in the writing process, <u>revision</u>.

Example 7–1

Look at how one student <u>expanded</u> a writing plan into a first draft.

WRITING PLAN

Subject: Child abuse
Purpose: To persuade reader of the danger of child abuse
Form: Report
Audience: Nursing assistants

Child abuse is a danger to children that results in harmful injury and even death. As nursing assistants, we have to be aware of the symptoms of child abuse. When we examine children who are repeatedly bruised, or accident prone, we should be suspicious. Neglecting to report cases when children are repeatedly being treated for broken bones could lead to greater injury. Child abuse affects children of all ages and crosses all economic groups. If we do not act on our suspicions because we want to protect the parents, the children will be <u>endangered</u>.

EXERCISE 7–1

Directions: As you read this first draft, think about the writing plan. Did the student stick to the writing plan? Yes ____ No ____. If you think changes were made, list the changes:

_____

_____

_____

_____

The student referred back to the collection of details in the map, list, or topic outline developed in the prewriting strategies in Chapter 6. This collection of details helps a writer turn the writing plan into a first draft.

EXERCISE 7-2

Directions: Look at the writing plan you developed in Chapter 6. Check the method you used to collect your details. Did you write:

- A map? _____
- A list? _____
- A topic outline? _____

EXERCISE 7-3

Directions: Use your writing plan and your map, list, or topic outline as your guide to write your first draft. Write freely. Get all your ideas on paper. Remember that you will have time to make changes during the next step in the writing process.

GETTING THE MAIN IDEAS ON PAPER

Did you write all your main ideas on your subject? Did you include all of the details that you collected? Did you choose to eliminate information or did you just forget to include it? Look back to your first step in the writing process. Reread your writing plan and your collection of details. Check your first draft against your prewriting strategies. See if there is anything you need to add to your first draft.

Example 7-2

Examine the student's first draft on the subject of child abuse. This student used the writing plan and map developed in Chapter 6 as a guide to write the first draft.

When the student checked the first draft against the writing plan it was evident that the subject, purpose, and audience followed the plan. However, the tone, or mood, of the draft did not seem appropriate for the chosen form, a report. It seemed that a report should be more detailed.

EXERCISE 7–4

Directions: Look again at the map of the student's collection of details from Chapter 6:

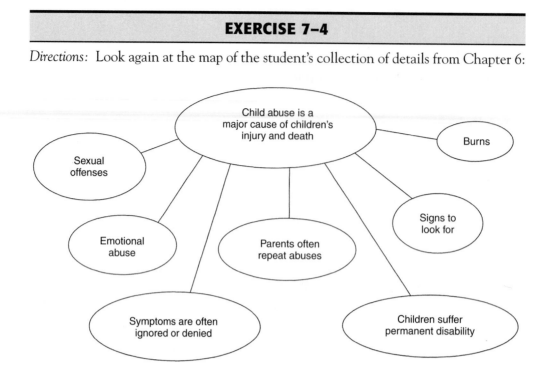

Were all of the details included? Yes _____ No _____. Are more specific details needed for a report? Yes _____ No _____. The student will have to make these decisions before revising this draft and handing in the final copy.

EXERCISE 7–5

Directions: Check your first draft against your writing plan and collection of details that you used as your guide. Did you follow your plan? Yes___ No ___. Did you change any of the following?

Subject _____

Purpose _____

Form _____

Audience _____

Did you include all of the information from your collection of details?

Yes _____ No _____.

Did you choose to change any information? Yes _____ No _____.

Did you forget to include any information? Yes _____ No _____.

Using your writing plan as a guide helps you to organize your information when you write your first draft.

ORGANIZING YOUR THINKING

While you are writing a first draft, it is helpful to try to organize your thinking. Think again about your purpose for writing. Do you want to **describe, explain, persuade,** or **narrate?**

Try to write freely while you organize your information according to purpose. When you are **describing,** use adjectives which arouse the senses. Will a reader be able to see, hear, feel, taste or smell when reading your writing? When you choose to **explain** something, you can give reasons and results. Hopefully, your readers will be able to <u>detect</u> a cause-effect relationship. If you compare or contrast things in your explanation, are you telling what something is like by letting the reader know how it is the same as or different from something else? You might choose to explain information by breaking it down into parts or by letting the reader know how something works. When you are writing to **persuade,** your purpose is to convince. Do you **slant** your writing? <u>Slanted</u> writing is writing that is deliberately chosen to sway a reader's opinion. Strong words are used to direct the reader to agree with the writer's opinion. When you are writing to **narrate,** you are telling a story. You might be telling about an experience you had or about an event that influenced you. When you are narrating a story, pay close attention to your <u>sequence</u> of events because logical order is important if a reader is to follow and understand your writing.

Example 7–3

The student who was writing about child abuse chose **persuasion** as a purpose. If you look at the draft, you can find the words that are slanted to convince the reader that child abuse is dangerous. Examine the slanted words which have been italicized in this student's first draft.

Child abuse is a *danger* to children that results in *harmful injury* and even *death.* As nursing assistants, we have to be aware of the symptoms of child abuse. When we examine children who are repeatedly *bruised,* or accident prone, we should be *suspicious. Neglecting* to report cases when children are repeatedly being treated for *broken bones* could lead to *greater injury.* Child abuse affects children of all ages and crosses all economic groups. If we do not act on our suspicions because we want to protect the parents, the children will be *endangered.*

EXERCISE 7–6

Directions: Look at your first draft. Check how you organized your information:

- **Describing** _____
- **Explaining** _____
- **Persuading** _____
- **Narrating** _____

EXERCISE 7–7

Directions: Read your first draft again. Circle any words that are examples of slanted writing. Explain why you chose these words to support your purpose in writing.

INCLUDING ALL THE PARTS

When you write your first draft, try to include all the necessary parts. Your writing should include a **beginning, middle,** and **ending.** Each part serves a purpose in your writing. Although you will be checking for these parts in your revision, it is helpful to think of them before you write your ideas.

The **beginning** should get your reader's attention and introduce your subject. The **middle** should support, explain, or describe your subject. The **ending** should summarize your main point and keep your reader thinking about your subject.

Example 7–4

Let's look for a **beginning, middle,** and **ending** in the student's first draft on the subject child abuse.

Child abuse is a danger to children that results in harmful injury and even death. As nursing assistants, we have to be aware of the symptoms of child abuse. When we examine children who are repeatedly bruised, or accident prone, we should be suspicious. Neglecting to report cases when children are repeatedly being treated for broken bones could lead to greater injury. Child abuse affects children of all ages and crosses all economic groups. If we do not act on our suspicions because we want to protect the parents, the children will be endangered.

The subject and the main idea about the subject → Child abuse is harmful
is introduced in the first sentence.
Sentences 2, 3 and 4 provide the details which → Symptoms
support the main idea.

Bruised
Accident
Suspicious
Broken bones
Injury
All ages and economic groups

The last sentence gives <u>emphasis</u> to the importance → Children endangered
of the main idea.

EXERCISE 7–8

Directions: Reread your first draft. Check to see if you have a **beginning, middle,** and **ending.** Underline the beginning and ending. Circle all the details in the middle that support the main idea.

FINISHING THE FIRST DRAFT

Your first draft isn't going to be perfect. Once you have all your main ideas on paper and have thought about the organization of your ideas, you are ready to revise your work. Check for your main ideas and details by looking for the 5Ws in your writing:

- **Who or what?**
- **What is the main point being made about the subject?**
- **When?**
- **Where?**
- **Why or how?**

If you have all the information you need, put your first draft down and take a break before you come back to take the next step in your writing—**revision.**

REVIEWING WRITING THE FIRST DRAFT

TO LEARN	USE THIS STRATEGY
To get started	Follow your writing plan and collection of details
To get your main ideas on paper	Check your writing plan and collection of details
To organize your thinking	Organize your writing according to your purpose: describe, explain, persuade or narrate
To include all the parts	Think about a beginning, middle, and ending as you write
To finish the first draft	Check that you have included all your main ideas by asking and answering the 5W questions

Chapter 8

Rewriting the Final Draft

LEARNING OBJECTIVES

In this chapter you will learn how to
• Follow a revising plan
• Use a computer to make revising easier
• Follow a plan for editing and proofreading
• Avoid trouble spots in your writing

VOCABULARY WORDS

These vocabulary words are important to your understanding the ideas in this chapter. These vocabulary words are underscored the first time they are used in the chapter. Read the list of words and definitions. Then check your understanding of these words before you read the chapter.

battered bruised.
choppy short sentence.
delete remove.
focused directed.
imperative essential.
mechanics punctuation, sentence style, word choice, capitalization, grammar.
presentation the appearance.
resistant tending to oppose.
tedious boring.
welts a lump on the body caused by a heavy blow.

VOCABULARY CHECK

Directions: Choose the vocabulary word that best fits into the sentence.

1. Marcy _____ her attention on her work.
2. Lewis was asked to _____ the unnecessary information from the proposal.
3. The _____ of Susie's writing had so many errors that it interfered with her message.
4. It is _____ that you finish your assignment before you take the test.
5. Don't be _____ to good advice.
6. Richard's story was so _____ we all stopped listening.
7. The _____ sentences in Maria's paper prevented a smooth reading.
8. The sloppy _____ of your paper will detract from the effort you put into the content.
9. The _____ child was taken to the hospital for treatment.
10. The _____ on the baby's back were not caused by a fall.

INTRODUCTION

After you have developed your writing plan and completed your first draft you are ready for the next step in the writing process. Remember, your first draft is not your final draft. You have to go through the steps of revising, editing, and proofreading before you have a final version of your paper.

Revising is the changes you make to improve your first draft. You will want to look at the main ideas and make some additions or cut some unnecessary details. You might want to change the order of your information. It helps to follow a plan when you are revising. Otherwise, you might not make all the needed improvements to your final draft.

FOLLOWING A PLAN FOR REVISING

You should follow this plan when you are revising your writing:

- Read the first draft several times.
- Think about the changes needed to improve your first draft. For example, ask yourself if you've included all the important ideas. Are any important details missing? Check to see if these ideas are clear, complete, and in the right order.
- Try to improve your writing by evaluating your own work. Look for the parts you want to keep. Look for the parts that need to be changed. You can use a revising checklist to help you evaluate your work and decide what changes need to be made to improve your first draft.

USING A REVISING CHECKLIST

The following checklist should help you to decide what to change as you revise your first draft. Ask yourself:

DID I	YES	NO
follow my writing plan?	_____	_____
clearly express my main idea?	_____	_____
support the main idea with enough details?	_____	_____
organize the details according to my purpose?	_____	_____
write a clear beginning, middle, and ending?	_____	_____
write the ideas in the correct order?	_____	_____
include unnecessary details?	_____	_____
repeat ideas?	_____	_____
fulfill my purpose in writing?	_____	_____

Answering the questions on the revising checklist will help you to examine the strengths and weaknesses of the first draft. You will now decide how to change your first draft to make it better.

Example 8–1

Let's take another look at the student's first draft on the subject of child abuse:

Child abuse is a danger to children that results in harmful injury and even death. As nursing assistants, we have to be aware of the symptoms of child abuse. When we examine children who are repeatedly bruised, or accident prone, we should be suspicious. Neglecting to report cases when children are repeatedly being treated for broken bones could lead to greater injury. Child abuse affects children of all ages and crosses all economic groups. If we do not act on our suspicions because we want to protect the parents, the children will be endangered.

This is how the student answered the question on the revising checklist:

DID I	YES	NO
follow my writing plan?	<u>Yes</u>, except more specific details are needed to fit the form of a report.	_____
clearly express my main idea?	_____	<u>No</u>, main point should be more directly stated.
support the main idea with enough details?	_____	<u>No</u>, more specific details were needed to make the report complete.
organize the details according to my purpose?	<u>Yes</u>, reasons were given to support conclusion.	_____
write a clear beginning, middle, and ending?	_____	<u>No</u>, middle needs to be more specific. Ending could be stronger.
write the ideas in the correct order?	<u>Yes</u>	_____
include unnecessary details?	_____	<u>No</u>
repeat ideas?	_____	<u>No</u>
fulfill my purpose in writing?	_____	<u>No</u>, conclusion has to be rewritten to fulfill purpose.

Example 8–2

The following is an example of the first revision:

Child abuse is a danger to children that may result in harmful injury and even death. As nursing assistants, we have to be aware of the symptoms of child abuse. When we examine children who are repeatedly bruised, or accident prone, we should be suspicious. Neglecting to report cases when children are repeatedly being treated for broken bones could lead to greater injury. Two weeks ago, a nine-year-old child was admitted to the hospital with a broken arm. Upon examination, several older bruises were discovered. This case is now being investigated by social services. This week, an infant was brought in with a head injury. The mother reported that the infant had fallen out of her highchair. However, this same mother brought in a toddler the week before with an arm pulled out of the socket. This toddler also had deep <u>welts</u> across the back and shoulders. The parent claimed not to know how the child got these welts. This case is also being looked into.

Child abuse affects children of all ages and crosses all economic groups.

If you have even the slightest evidence that a child is being abused, report the case to social services. If we do not act on our suspicions because we want to protect the parents, the children will be endangered.

Excercise 8–1

Directions: Reread your first draft. Read the revising check list. Answer the questions. Make the needed changes to your first draft.

After you have revised your first draft, look at your revision and make sure that you have made all the needed changes. Is there anything else that you would like to add or <u>delete</u>? Is your subject <u>focused</u>? Does your conclusion sum up the information? Are all the important details included? Take another look at your writing. You may have to make more changes. Sometimes several revisions are needed before a writer is satisfied. Remember not to worry about spelling and <u>mechanics</u> during the revising stage. When you are revising, you are concentrating on the organization of your main ideas and important details.

Example 8–3

Read the student's second revision of the report on child abuse.

Child abuse is a danger to children that may result in harmful injury and even death. As nursing assistants, we have to be aware of the symptoms of child abuse. When we examine children who are repeatedly bruised, or accident prone, we should be suspicious. Neglecting to report cases when children are repeatedly being treated for broken bones could lead to greater injury. Two weeks ago, a nine-year-old child was admitted to the hospital with a broken arm. Upon examination, several older bruises were discovered. This case is now being investigated by social services. This week, an infant was brought in with a head injury. The mother reported that the infant had fallen out of her highchair. However, this same mother brought in a toddler the week before with an arm pulled out of the socket. This toddler also had deep welts across the back and shoulders. The parent claimed not to know how the child got these welts. Both children had been <u>battered</u>. This case is also being looked into.

Child abuse affects children of all ages and crosses all economic groups. In the last month, two of the seven reported cases of child abuse were from upper-middle class homes with both parents.

If you have even the slightest evidence that a child is being abused, report the case to social services. If we do not act on our suspicions because we want to protect the parents, the children will be endangered. Therefore, it is <u>imperative</u> that you report all cases of suspected child abuse to the social service agency.

EXERCISE 8–2

Directions: Read the second revision. Underline any additions you notice. Did the student make any other changes? Yes ___ No ___. Look at the revision checklist again. Did the student make all the needed changes? Yes ___ No ___. Explain your answer.

EXERCISE 8–3

Directions: Read your revision. Do you need to make any further changes? If so, revise your paper again. Make all the changes that you think are needed before you go on to the next step in the revision process, editing and proofreading.

It may take several revisions before you make all the changes that you think are needed to improve your writing. Students are often underlined resistant to revising their papers. Many students make the mistake of trying to avoid the revising step in the writing process. They hand in their first draft as their final draft, and then they are disappointed when their papers receive poor grades.

Students are reluctant to revise papers for many reasons. They mistakenly think that good papers can be written in one step, or they do not want to put in the time needed to make the necessary improvements.

Many students have found that a computer helps them go through the steps of revising. If you don't own a computer, find out if your school and library have computers you can use.

USING A COMPUTER TO HELP WITH REVISING

Many students use the computer from the first step in the writing process—planning—until they hand in their final draft. Other students prefer to do their planning and first drafts on paper and then type their work on the computer to do the revising and editing that is needed before turning in the final draft.

Word processing programs help you use the computer to add ideas and move sentences and even whole pages around. Using a word processor makes revising less tedious. Writing becomes less of a chore and more exciting. Students actually enjoy moving their ideas around. It's fun to see the changes as they appear on the computer screen. Editing is also easier with the computer. Computer programs have spell checks that scan for spelling errors and grammar checks that point out mechanical problems with sentences.

Using a computer will make it much easier for you to make the changes needed to improve your writing.

FOLLOWING A PLAN FOR EDITING AND PROOFREADING

When you have finished revising the ideas in your paper, you are ready for another step in the writing process, editing and proofreading. During editing and proofreading, you make your final changes. You carefully check your writing for errors in spelling and mechanics. You should follow this plan for editing and proofreading your writing: Check

- sentences to determine whether they are smooth or <u>choppy</u>.
- for errors in spelling, punctuation, and grammar.
- your choice of words.
- the <u>presentation</u> of your finished copy.
- your paper one last time to make sure that you have corrected any mistakes.

USING A CHECKLIST FOR EDITING AND PROOFREADING

The following checklist should help you to edit and proofread your writing. Ask yourself:

DID I	YES	NO
write clear and complete sentences?	____	____
use sentence variety?	____	____
write sentences of different lengths?	____	____
capitalize and punctuate correctly?	____	____
choose vivid, specific words?	____	____
check for repetition of words?	____	____
check for subject-verb agreement?	____	____
check for pronoun agreement?	____	____
check for verb tense?	____	____
check spelling errors?	____	____

The questions on this editing and proofreading checklist will help you to make the final corrections needed to improve your writing.

Example 8–4

Let's reread the student's second revision of the report on child abuse:

Child abuse is a danger to children that may result in harmful injury and even death. As nursing assistants, we have to be aware of the symptoms of child abuse. When we examine children who are repeatedly bruised, or accident prone, we should be suspicious. Neglecting to report cases when children are repeatedly being treated for broken bones could lead to greater injury. Two weeks ago, a nine-year-old child was admitted to the hospital with a broken arm. Upon examination, several older bruises were discovered. This case is now being investigated by social services. This week, an infant was brought in with a head injury. The mother reported that the infant had fallen out of her highchair. However, this same mother brought in a toddler the week before with an arm pulled out of the socket. This toddler also had deep welts across the back and shoulders. The parent claimed not to know how the child got these welts. Both children had been battered. This case is also being looked into.

Child abuse affects children of all ages and crosses all economic groups. In the last month, two of the seven reported cases of child abuse were from upper-middle class homes with both parents.

If you have even the slightest evidence that a child is being abused, report the case to social services. If we do not act on our suspicions because we want to protect the parents, the children will be endangered. Therefore, it is <u>imperative</u> that you report all cases of suspected child abuse to the social service agency.

This is how the student answered the questions on the editing and proofreading checklist.

- Did I write clean and complete sentences? *Yes.*
- Did I use sentence variety? *Sentences 7 and 8 begin the same way.*
- Did I choose vivid, specific words? *Word choice could be improved.*
- Did I use sentences of different lengths? *Yes.*
- Did I avoid repetitions? *No. The words abuse, also, all, repeatedly, and suspected were used too often.*
- Did I capitalize and punctuate correctly? *An exclamation point could be used instead of a period for emphasis. Change Social to lower case.*
- Did I check for subject-verb agreement? *Yes.*
- Did I check for pronoun persons? *No. The report should be kept in second person.*
- Did I check for verb tense? *Yes.*
- Did I check for spelling errors? *Yes.*

Once you have decided on the changes that need to be made, you can use certain tools to help you. You can use spell check and grammar check in your computer word processing program. You can also use a dictionary to check spelling, meaning, and parts of speech and a thesaurus to give you choices of words with similar meanings to avoid repetition. Many computer word processing programs include a dictionary and thesaurus.

LEARNING SOME BASIC SYMBOLS FOR PROOFREADING

You can use proofreading symbols to help you mark up your revised paper so that you can make the final changes. Learning these symbols will also help you to understand your instructor's corrections of your writing.

Some common proofreading symbols are

agr agreement.
cap capitalization.
frag sentence fragment.
gram grammar.
nc not clear.
¶ paragraph
p punctuation.

R repetitions.
sp misspelled word.
RO run-on sentence.
TS topic sentence
u usage.
wc word choice.

Example 8–5

Read the student's final draft of the report on child abuse.

Child abuse is a danger to children that may result in harmful injury and even death. As nursing assistants, you have to be aware of the symptoms of child abuse. When you examine children who are frequently bruised, or accident prone, you should be wary. Neglecting to report cases when children are repeatedly being treated for broken bones could lead to greater injury. Two weeks ago, a nine-year-old child was admitted to the hospital with a broken arm. Upon examination, several older bruises were discovered. Social services is now investigating this case. This week, an infant was brought in with a head injury. The mother reported that the infant had fallen out of her highchair. However, this same mother brought in a toddler the week before with an arm pulled out of the socket. In addition, the toddler had deep welts across the upper back and shoulders. The parent claimed not to know how the child got these welts. Both children had been battered. Social services will explore this matter further.

Child abuse affects children of all ages and crosses every economic group. In the last month, two of the seven reported cases of child abuse were from upper-middle class homes with both parents. If you have even the slightest evidence that a child is being harmed, the case should be reported to social services. If you do not act on your suspicions because you want to protect the parents, the children will be endangered. Therefore, it is imperative that you report all cases of assumed child abuse to the social service agency.

EXERCISE 8–4

Directions: Use the editing and proofreading checklist and the proofreading symbols as guides to correct your revision. Write your final draft.

PREPARING THE PRESENTATION

The presentation, or appearance, of your paper is a critical part of the writing process. Whether you write or type your paper, your work should be neat, well spaced, and easy to read. In writing, one cannot separate form from content. A finished paper with a good presentation is an essential part of the writing process.

AVOIDING TROUBLE SPOTS IN WRITING

When you are proofreading your paper, keep in mind certain areas in which students make errors. If you are aware of these problem areas in writing, you can correct your mistakes before you hand in your final paper.

SPELLING

You can avoid making spelling mistakes by learning and applying a few spelling rules.

Some Common Spelling Rules

- **Words ending in "Y":** When you write the plurals of words that end in **y**, change **y** to **i** and add **es.** If the word ends in **ey**, just add **s.**
  baby, babies   turkey, turkeys
- **Consonant Ending:** When you add an ending like **ed** or **ing** to a one-syllable word with a short vowel, the final consonant is usually doubled.
  hop, hopping   tip, tipped
- **"I" Before "E":** **I** before **e** except after **c** or when rhyming with **say** as in **neighbor** and **weigh.**
  belief, conceit, sleigh
- **Silent "E":** If a word ends with a silent **e,** drop the **e** before adding an ending that begins with a vowel. Do not drop the **e** when the ending begins with a consonant.
  hope, hoping, hopeful

Commonly Misspelled Words

You should learn the following words that students often misspell:

Absence	Dilemma	Height
Absent	Disease	Helpful
Accept	Dissatisfied	Hospital
Accident	Dying	
Accommodate		Illegal
Accurate	Embarrassed	Immigrant
Across	Environment	Independent
Advise	Excellence	Intelligence
Already	Exercise	Interfere
Analyze	Exhaust	Itinerary
Apologize	Extremely	
Attendance		Jeopardize
	Feasible	Judgment
Belief	Foreign	
Benefit	Fragile	Knowledge
Benefited	Friend	
Business	Fulfill	Laboratory
		Leisure
Characteristic	Government	
Committee	Grievance	Maintenance
Competition	Guarantee	Medicine
Convenience	Guardian	
Cooperate		Necessary
Criticism	Handicapped	Neighborhood
	Handkerchief	Neither
Decision	Harass	Nuclear
Dependent	Hazardous	
		Occasion
		Occur

Omitted

Operate

Opinion

Pamphlet

Persuade

Physical

Physically

Preferred

Prejudice

Professor

Pronunciation

Psychology

Qualitative

Questionnaire

Receipt

Recognize

Recommend

Recurrence

Reference

Remember

Responsibilities

Safety

Schedule

Secretary

Separate

Significant

Suggest

Supervisory

Sympathize

Tedious

Temperature

Temporarily

Tendency

Tomorrow

Tragedy

Transferred

Traveling

Ultimately

Unconscious

Unfortunately

Unnecessary

Vehicle

Violence

Voluntary

Waive

Weigh

Welfare

Witnessed

Yield

Zeros

EXERCISE 8–5

Directions: Choose the correct spelling of the following words:

1. coppyed copied coppied
2. poked pokked pokd
3. neighbor nieghbor nieighbor
4. guardain gardian guardian
5. handkercheif hankerchief handkerchief
6. easier easyier easyer
7. hopeless hoppless hopeles
8. judgement judgment juddgment
9. temperture temperature temparature
10. dryed dried dryied

Words Often Confused

Read over the following commonly misused words. This list should help you find the right words to use in your writing.

accept to receive.
except other than.

allowed permitted.
aloud with a speaking voice.

already previously.
all ready completely ready.

capital the seat of government.
   chief.
   accumulated wealth.

capitol a building that usually
   houses some part of government.

choose to select.
chose selected.

council a group called together for
   certain tasks.
counsel advise.
   to give advice.

desert a dry region.
   to leave.
dessert the final course of a meal.

it's the contraction meaning "it is."
its the possessive form of "it."

loose free from restrictions.
lose to misplace.
   to fail to win.

principal a school administrator.
   most important.
principle a rule.

stationary a fixed position.
stationery writing paper.

than compares two things.
then tells when.

their possessive form of they.
there indicates place or direction.
they're a contraction meaning "they are."

to indicates direction.
too also.
   very.
two the number "2."

who's the contraction meaning
   "who is."
whose the possessive form of "who."

you're the contraction meaning
   "you are."
your the possessive form of "you."

EXERCISE 8–6

Directions: Choose the correct word in each sentence:

1. _____ (Who's, Whose) picking you up from school today?

2. I have to order new _____ (stationary, stationery) to write my thank you notes.

3. Mr. Miller is the _____ (principal, principle) of my school.

4. Yesterday the team _____ (choose, chose) Allan to be the captain.

5. Everyone _____ (accept, except) Elizabeth was invited to the party.

6. _____ (Their, There, They're) going to be late for the movie.

7. Are you _____ (allowed, aloud) to take out three books from the library?

8. These suitcases are _____ (to, too, two) heavy for me to carry.

9. Chocolate cake is my favorite _____ (desert, dessert).

10. Try not to _____ (loose, lose).

Sentence Errors

A sentence is made up of a subject and verb and expresses a complete thought. Check for sentence errors. Some common errors are sentence fragments and run-on sentences.

A fragment is a group of words that does not make a complete sentence.

Example: Thinks he can win.

This fragment is missing a subject. You can correct this fragment by adding a subject.

Corrected Sentence: My brother thinks he can win.

A run-on sentence is when two sentences are joined without punctuation or a connecting word.

Example: I thought he would never leave he just kept talking.

Corrected Sentence: I thought he would never leave. He just kept talking.

EXERCISE 8–7

Directions: Label each group of words as *fragment, run-on,* or *correct sentence.*

1. To fly a plane. _____

2. Many infections can be prevented. _____

3. Because the virus wasn't treated correctly. _____

4. This test is too difficult I should have studied harder. _____

5. I am allergic to chocolate it makes me break out in hives. _____

6. Call the supervisor if you have a problem with this patient. _____

7. During the intermission. _____

8. People were inoculated. _____

9. The orderly brought ice-cream to the tonsillectomy patient she enjoyed it.

_____

10. Hopeful for a complete recovery. _____

Parts of Speech

Learning the parts of speech will help you to know how to use words correctly in a sentence. Read over the following chart to learn how to use the parts of speech.

PARTS OF SPEECH	USE	EXAMPLES
noun	names	pen, Lewis
pronoun	taking the place of a noun	them, us, herself
adjective	describes a noun or pronoun	red, tallest
verb	action, linking, helping	watched, is, has been writing
adverb	describes a verb, an adjective, or another adverb	slowly, better
preposition	relates a noun or pronoun to another word; begins a phrase	among, around, on
conjunction	joins words	and, but, or
interjection	shows strong feeling	Ouch!

EXERCISE 8–8

Directions: Write the correct part of speech of each italicized word in the following paragraph.

Marcia was having difficulty studying *for* her midterm exams. *Her family* and *work* responsibilities *were interfering* with the hours she needed for study. Studying, working, *and* child care were hard to juggle. Marcia knew she could do *better in* school if she had more time for herself. Sometimes, she felt like crying *"help!"*

Agreement

Pronouns

Pronouns must agree in person and number with the words they replace.

Example: John told *Sonya* and *Mary* to meet him at work.

He told *them* to meet him at work.

Example: *Sylvia* instructed *the employees* on how to operate *the computer*. *She* instructed *them* on how to operate *it*.

Subjects and Verbs

Subjects and verbs should agree in number. If the subject is singular, the verb should be singular. If the subject is plural, the verb should be plural. In the following examples the subject is in italic type and the verb is in boldface type.

Example: *Mindy and Helen* **were** absent.

Example: *Either* of the doctors **is** qualified to perform the surgery.

The following words take a singular verb:

Anyone	Everybody	One
Everyone	Each	Someone
Anybody	Either	Neither

EXERCISE 8–9

Directions: Choose the right answer for each of these sentences.

1. Does anyone _____ (live, lives) here?

2. He and I _____ (was, were) at home.

3. One of my friends _____ (is, are) coming to visit.

4. Elijah took _____ (his, him) car to the station.

5. Jackie and Matthew were hoping _____ (they, he) could get a ride to the game.

6. When the medicine expires _____ (it, its) is no longer effective.

7. Everybody _____ (expects, expect) to pass the course.

8. Katherine left _____ (her, hers) book at home.

9. The patient left _____ (his, him) insurance form at home.

10. Antonio _____ (follow, follows) instructions correctly.

Capitalization

Capitalize

- the first word of a sentence
- proper nouns and adjectives

Example: *Celena* traveled to *England* and enjoyed touring the *English* countryside.

Punctuation

Read the following chart to learn how to use punctuation correctly.

.	Period	End of sentence that makes a statement, command, or request
		After abbreviated title or initial
?	Question mark	End of sentence that asks a question
!	Exclamation mark	End of sentence that shows emotion
,	Comma	Items in a series
		In dates, addresses, and numbers
		After introductory expressions
		Around nonessential material
		To set off interruptions
		In direct address
'	Apostrophe	To form the possessive of singular and plural nouns
		In contractions
;	Semicolon	Between two closely related independent clauses unless they are joined by the connecting words (and, but, nor, yet, or, for, so)
:	Colon	After a complete statement when a list or long quotation follows
—	Dash	To show a change of thought or emphasis
" "	Quotation marks	Around the exact words of a speaker
		The name of a short story, poem, essay, or TV program

EXERCISE 8–10

Directions: Put the correct capitalization and punctuation in the following paragraph.

Rosa is taking english lessons so that she will be able to get a better job. She is hoping to improve her skills in reading writing and conversation when she finishes this course she will be able to enter a community college. Will this course give her skills she needs to succeed. She will have to meet the following requirements taking notes, understanding lectures and comprehending her textbooks. rosa hopes to become a technician when she moves to philadelphia in two years.

REVIEWING REWRITING THE FINAL DRAFT

TO LEARN	USE THIS STRATEGY
Make necessary changes to your first draft	Follow a plan for revising
Decide what changes are necessary	Use a revising checklist
Make additional changes	Reread your revision
Make revising easier	Use a word-processing program
Make the needed changes in spelling and mechanics	Use an editing and proofreading checklist
Mark your paper so you will remember to make all your changes to prepare your final draft	Use proofreading symbols
Prepare the final presentation	Remember that form cannot be separated from content
Avoid trouble spots in your writing	Review some basic rules and do practice exercises in spelling, sentences, parts of speech, agreement, capitalization, and punctuation

UNIT III

MATHEMATICS STRATEGIES

You may be one of many students who are anxious at the thought of doing mathematics in the health sciences. This unit has been written to ease this anxiety and to teach you the strategies for solving basic math functions. Chapter 9, Learning Computation Skills, will teach you the mathematical foundation of multiplying and dividing whole numbers. Also, you will learn the strategies for solving fraction, decimal, percentage, ratio, and proportion problems. Chapter 10, Understanding Algebra, Geometry, and the Metric System, will go one gentle step further and teach you the basics of algebra, geometry, and performing conversions in the metric system. Unit 3 will conclude with Chapter 11, Solving Word Problems. In this chapter, you will learn how to solve word problems by identifying the various terms that will indicate the operation to perform in word problems. Although Unit 3, Mathematics Strategies, is not intended to be a complete course in math, it is hoped that it will provide a good reintroduction to math. Once you finish all the exercises in this unit, your confidence should be strong and your interest should be sparked for learning more.

Chapter
9

Learning Computation Skills

LEARNING OBJECTIVES

In this chapter you will learn how to
- Memorize multiplication and division facts
- Solve problems using fractions, decimals, percentages, ratios and proportions

VOCABULARY WORDS

The following vocabulary words are important to your understanding of the ideas in this chapter. These vocabulary words are underscored the first time they are used in the chapter. Read the list of words and definitions. Then check your understanding of these words before you read the chapter.

caret a punctuation mark that shows in what place an item will be inserted.

common belonging to or shared by two or more mathematical entities.

comparison showing similarities of two or more items.

conversion the act of changing or transforming.

denominator the part of a fraction below the line that signifies division.

diagonal passing from the upper left to the lower right or the upper right to the lower left.

numerator the part of a fraction above the line that signifies division.

reverse to go in an opposite direction.

typical having the nature or being part of a type.

values numerical quantities.

VOCABULARY CHECK

Directions: Choose the vocabulary word that best fits into the sentence.

1. The checks in her wallet had different _____.

2. It was bright and sunny; it was a _____ summer day.

3. The children will march in one direction; then they will _____ their march to a different direction.

4. The top part of a fraction is the _____.

5. The stripes did not go up and down or side to side; they went on a_____.

6. The bottom part of a fraction is the _____.

7. He checked a _____ chart to change Fahrenheit into Celsius.

8. All the fish looked alike so they were considered a _____ type.

9. He left out the word "medicine" so he wrote a _____ and inserted the word in the proper place.

10. The _____ of the twins showed that they were identical.

MULTIPLICATION

Multiplication is the fast way of adding similar numbers over and over again. You can recognize a multiplication problem when you see the × sign. To do multiplication problems well, you must memorize the multiplication tables. As an example, the multiplication table for 3 looks like the following:

$$0 \times 3 = 0 \qquad 7 \times 3 = 21$$
$$1 \times 3 = 3 \qquad 8 \times 3 = 24$$
$$2 \times 3 = 6 \qquad 9 \times 3 = 27$$
$$3 \times 3 = 9 \qquad 10 \times 3 = 30$$
$$4 \times 3 = 12 \qquad 11 \times 3 = 33$$
$$5 \times 3 = 15 \qquad 12 \times 3 = 36$$
$$6 \times 3 = 18$$

You can create similar multiplication tables for any number. However, there is a better strategy for learning the multiplication tables—making and learning the multiplication chart (see Table 9–1).

The method for using this chart is as follows:

- You are asked to figure out how many ounces of medicine Ms. Grande takes per week. You know that she takes 3 ounces a day.
- In your mind you see the problem as $7 \times 3 = ?$, where 7 stands for the number of days in a week and 3 stands for the number of ounces of medicine Ms. Grande takes per day.
- In the top shaded row, put your right finger on the number 7.
- In the shaded column to the left, put your left finger on the number 3.
- Slowly move your right finger down and your left finger to the right until they meet. The number at which both fingers meet is the correct answer.
- "21 oz." is the answer to this problem.

TABLE 9–1 Multiplication Chart

×	1	2	3	4	5	6	7	8	9	10	11	12
1	1	2	3	4	5	6	7	8	9	10	11	12
2	2	4	6	8	10	12	14	16	18	20	22	24
3	3	6	9	12	15	18	21	24	27	30	33	36
4	4	8	12	16	20	24	28	32	36	40	44	48
5	5	10	15	20	25	30	35	40	45	50	55	60
6	6	12	18	24	30	36	42	48	54	60	66	72
7	7	14	21	28	35	42	49	56	63	70	77	84
8	8	16	24	32	40	48	56	64	72	80	88	96
9	9	18	27	36	45	54	63	72	81	90	99	108
10	10	20	30	40	50	60	70	80	90	100	110	120
11	11	22	33	44	55	66	77	88	99	110	121	132
12	12	24	36	48	60	72	84	96	108	120	132	144

Although a multiplication chart is very handy, it does not substitute for learning the tables by heart. Memorizing the multiplication tables until you know them as well as your name will make your personal and student life easier. To help you learn the tables, try making flash cards or find a computer program that will make the learning task enjoyable.

DIVISION

Like multiplication, you use division to solve many common, daily arithmetic problems. You can write division problems two ways:

$$10 \div 2 = 5$$

In this example the number 10 is divided by 2. In other words, you always divide the number after the sign into the number that goes before the sign. The second way to write division problems looks like this:

$$2\overline{)10}^{5}$$

In this example, you divide the number that is inside the box by the number that is outside the box. If you have learned your multiplication tables well, you will have an easier time with division. You may have noticed in the first example that if you read the problem from right to left, it reads like a multiplication problem. Consider the following:

- Mr. Sheldon, a medical secretary, was asked to split a $3000 bonus among the three employees working in Dr. Joseph's office.
- Mr. Sheldon knows that $1000 \times 3 = 3000$.
- He reverses the procedure and divided 3000 by 3.
- Each employee will get $1000.

If you learn the multiplication tables thoroughly, you will be able to do more complicated multiplication and division problems.

EXERCISE 9–1

Directions: Spend some time learning the multiplication chart (Table 9–1). Then fill in the chart at the top of p. 133. You may want to memorize one table at a time and then fill in the chart as you learn that table. Remember that learning the multiplication tables by heart will help you with both multiplication and division problems.

×	1	2	3	4	5	6	7	8	9	10	11	12
1												
2												
3												
4												
5												
6												
7												
8												
9												
10												
11												
12												

FRACTIONS

Fractions represent parts of a whole. You go to school 5 days out of 7 days. When this is written as a fraction, it looks like this:

$$\frac{5}{7}$$

In this example the number 5 on top is called the <u>numerator</u>. The numerator tells you how many parts of the whole. The number 7 on the bottom is called the <u>denominator</u>. The denominator tells you how many parts make up a whole.

This example of a fraction is called a **proper fraction**. A proper fraction is when the numerator is smaller than the denominator and has a value less than 1.

Consider this next fraction:

$$\frac{4}{2}$$

This is an example of an **improper fraction**. When the numerator is larger than the denominator, you have an improper fraction.

Sometimes you may see a whole number written with a fraction next to it. It will look like this:

$$13\frac{6}{12}$$

This is called a **mixed number**.

Reducing to the Lowest Term

Sometimes when working with fractions it is necessary to reduce them to their lowest terms. This means dividing the numerator and the denominator by the same number until you cannot go any further. Study the following problem:

$$\frac{50}{100}$$

- What number is needed to divide both the 50 and 100 so that the answer comes out evenly?
- Try 25. 50 divided by 25 is 2. 100 divided by 25 is 4. The answer so far looks like this:

$$\frac{2}{4}$$

- Is it still possible to reduce this fraction? Is there still another number that can be divided equally into both the 2 and the 4?
- Try 2: 2 goes into 2 once; 2 goes into 4 twice. The answer now is:

$$\frac{1}{2}$$

The lowest term for

$$\frac{50}{100}$$

is

$$\frac{1}{2}$$

Raising to a Higher Term

- Similarly, any fraction can be changed to a higher term by multiplying both the numerator and the denominator by the same number.

$$\frac{9}{18} = \frac{27}{54}$$

$$9 \times 3 = 27 \text{ and } 18 \times 3 = 54$$

Adding and Subtracting Fractions

To add and subtract with fractions that have the same denominator, you add or subtract only the numerator and copy the <u>common</u> denominator to finish the problem.

$$\frac{5}{11} + \frac{3}{11} = \frac{8}{11}$$

$$\frac{9}{64} - \frac{1}{64} = \frac{8}{64}$$

However, if the denominators are different, you need to find the lowest common denominator. The lowest common denominator is the smallest number that can be divided evenly by the denominators of all the fractions in the problem. For example:

$$\frac{2}{3} \qquad\qquad \frac{5}{6} \qquad\qquad \frac{3}{9}$$

- Think of the smallest number that can be divided evenly by 3, 6, 9.

$$3 \times 6 = 18 \qquad 6 \times 3 = 18 \qquad 9 \times 2 = 18$$

Or

$$18 \div 3 = 6 \qquad 18 \div 6 = 3 \qquad 18 \div 9 = 2$$

18 is the lowest common denominator. The problem now looks like this:

$$\frac{(2)}{18} \qquad\qquad \frac{(5)}{18} \qquad\qquad \frac{(3)}{18}$$

- To finish the problem you must take one more important step. **Whatever you do to the denominator you must do to the numerator**.
- In the first fraction, you multiplied 3 by 6 to get the lowest common denominator of 18. Now you must do the same to the numerator 2. $2 \times 6 = 12$. The fraction is now

$$\frac{12}{18}$$

- In the second fraction you multiplied the denominator 6 by 3 to get the lowest common denominator of 18. Now you must do the same to the numerator 5. $5 \times 3 = 15$. The fraction is now

$$\frac{15}{18}$$

- In the third fraction you multiplied the denominator 9 by 2 to get the lowest common denominator of 18. Now you must do the same to the numerator 3. $3 \times 2 = 6$. The fraction is now

$$\frac{6}{18}$$

The fractions now look like this:

$$\frac{12}{18} \qquad\qquad \frac{15}{18} \qquad\qquad \frac{6}{18}$$

- These fractions are now ready to be added or subtracted.

Multiplying Fractions

To multiply fractions you simply multiply the numerators and then the denominators. For example:

$$\frac{4}{7} \times \frac{10}{10} = \frac{40}{10}$$

If you are working with mixed numbers, it is important to change them into improper fractions before multiplying or dividing. Look at the following:

$$2\frac{4}{8}$$

- To change this mixed number into an improper fraction, first multiply the denominator by the whole number.

$$8 \times 2 = 16$$

- Next add the numerator of 4 to the 16.

$$16 + 4 = 20$$

- Finally copy the original denominator so the fraction now looks like this:

$$\frac{20}{8}$$

- The mixed number has now been changed to an improper fraction.

Dividing Fractions

To divide fractions, you do the following two steps:

$$\frac{4}{16} \div \frac{5}{15}$$

First you <u>reverse</u> the second fraction. In other words, the 15 becomes the numerator and the 5 becomes the denominator.

$$\frac{15}{5}$$

Then you change the division sign to a multiplication sign and multiply the numerators and then the denominators to get the answer.

$$\frac{4}{16} \times \frac{15}{5} = \frac{60}{80} = \frac{3}{4}$$

Sometimes, if the numbers are large, you may want to reduce them in a multiplication or division problem. Remember to work on a <u>diagonal</u> across the signs.

$$\frac{10}{20} \times \frac{5}{40} \times \frac{1}{10}$$

$$\frac{\overset{1}{\cancel{10}}}{\underset{4}{\cancel{20}}} \times \frac{\overset{1}{\cancel{5}}}{40} \times \frac{1}{\underset{1}{\cancel{10}}} =$$

$$\frac{1}{4} \times \frac{1}{40} \times \frac{1}{1} = \frac{1}{160}$$

EXERCISE 9–2

Directions: Do the following fraction problems. Pay careful attention to the signs so that you perform the correct function. Remember to find the lowest common denominators if necessary and change any mixed numbers to improper fractions.

1. Reduce $\dfrac{12}{48}$

2. Determine the missing numerator: $\dfrac{2}{3} = \dfrac{?}{36}$

3. Change to an improper fraction: $9\dfrac{2}{14} =$

4. $\dfrac{9}{11} - \dfrac{7}{11} =$

5. $\dfrac{4}{28} + \dfrac{9}{28} + \dfrac{14}{28} =$

6. $\dfrac{1}{3} \times \dfrac{1}{2} =$

7. $\dfrac{1}{3} \div \dfrac{1}{2}$

8. $\dfrac{5}{14} \times \dfrac{7}{25} =$

9. $4\dfrac{8}{10} \div \dfrac{4}{5} =$

10. $2\dfrac{2}{4} \times 1\dfrac{5}{20}$

DECIMALS

Decimal numbers are similar to fractions. They both describe parts of a whole number. However, there are two differences between decimals and fractions. The first difference is that denominators of decimals can be only 10, 100, 1000, etc. The second difference is that a decimal point or period is used to separate the whole number from the fraction. In the following example, note the difference between decimals and fractions of the same number.

$$\dfrac{2}{10} = 0.2$$

$$\dfrac{80}{100} = 0.80$$

$$\dfrac{425}{1000} = 0.425$$

$$\dfrac{734}{10000} = 7.0034$$

The way you read a decimal is determined by how many numbers are to the right of the decimal point. The first example, 0.2, is read "two tenths." The second example, 0.80, is read "eighty hundredths." The third example, 0.425, is read "four hundred twenty-five thousandths," And the last example, 7.0034 is read "seven **and** thirty-four ten thousandths."

Adding and Subtracting Decimals

When you add or subtract decimals, it is necessary to write the problem so that all the decimal points are lined up in a straight row. Then add or subtract decimal numbers the same way you would add or subtract whole numbers.

$$\begin{array}{r} 4.258 \\ 9.636 \\ \underline{13.894} \end{array} \qquad \begin{array}{r} 90.58 \\ 82.21 \\ \underline{8.37} \end{array}$$

If you are adding or subtracting decimals, use zeros to fill in the places without a number after you align the decimal points.

$$\begin{array}{r} 21.55 \\ +62.2\mathbf{0} \\ \hline \end{array} \qquad \begin{array}{r} 21.55 \\ 62.2\mathbf{0} \\ \underline{83.75} \end{array} \qquad \begin{array}{r} 9.4707 \\ -4.26\mathbf{00} \\ \hline \end{array} \qquad \begin{array}{r} 9.4707 \\ 4.26\mathbf{00} \\ \underline{5.2107} \end{array}$$

Multiplying Decimals

When you multiply decimal numbers, multiply the same way you would with whole numbers. Then count all the numbers to the right of the decimal point in both rows of numbers in the problem. Put the decimal point that number of places in the answer.

$$\begin{array}{r} 0.798 \\ \times 6.4 \\ \hline 5.1072 \end{array}$$

(3 numbers to right of decimal point)
(1 number to right of decimal point)
(4 numbers to right of decimal point)

Dividing Decimals

Dividing decimal numbers is similar to dividing whole numbers. If the number outside the box is a whole number, place the decimal point in the answer in the same decimal place as the number inside the box.

$$4\overline{)0.8}^{\,0.2}$$

If the number outside the box is a decimal, change this decimal number to a whole number by moving the decimal point to the right of the last number. Use a <u>caret</u> (^) to show the new place of the decimal. If the number inside the box is also a decimal number, move the decimal point the same amount of numbers as you did the outside number. Also use a caret to show you have moved the decimal point. If necessary add zeros to get the same number of decimal places.

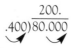

$$.400\overline{)80.000}^{\,200.}$$

Notice that the decimal point in the answer is placed exactly over the new position of the decimal point of the number inside the box.

Changing Decimals to Fractions

To change a decimal to a fraction, write the numbers in the decimal as the numerator and write the name of the decimal (tenths, hundredths, thousandths, etc.) as the denominator. Reduce the fraction if necessary.

$$0.50 = \frac{50}{100} = \frac{1}{2}$$

Changing Fractions to Decimals

To change a fraction to a decimal, divide the numerator by the denominator. The dividing line of a fraction means "divided by." To divide the numerator by the denominator, it will be necessary to add a decimal point and one or more zeros to the numerator. Carry the decimal point up to the answer.

$$\frac{1}{2} \qquad\qquad\qquad \begin{array}{r} 0.5 \\ 2\overline{)1.0} \end{array}$$

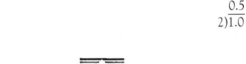

EXERCISE 9–3

Directions: Solve the following decimal problems.

Add the following decimals:

a. 5.439 + 7.63 + 1.257 =

b. 0.428 + 0.029 + 8.35 =

Subtract the following decimals:

c. 21.719 – 5.83 =

d. 103.8 – 62.45 =

Multiply the following decimals:

e. 943.27 × 0.5 =

f. 1.3294 × 0.566 =

Divide the following decimals:

g. 70 ÷ 0.25 =

h. 160 ÷ 0.40 =

Change the following decimals to fractions. Reduce the fractions if necessary.

i. 0.020   0.8   0.45

Change the following fractions to decimals:

j. $\frac{4}{5}$ $\frac{6}{80}$ $\frac{50}{250}$

PERCENTAGES

Percentage numbers, like fractions and decimals, represent a part of the whole. The percentage represents hundredths and is indicated by the percent sign (%). Thus 47 hundredths can be written as

$$\frac{47}{100}, 0.47, \text{ or } 47\%$$

When doing percentage problems, you should change the percentage number to either a fraction or a decimal number and then solve the problem. Table 9–2 is a <u>conversion</u> chart of some of the more common percentages.

Changing Percentages to Fractions

To change a percentage to a fraction, use the number in the percentage as the numerator and put 100 as the denominator. Reduce the fraction if necessary.

$$35\% = \frac{35}{100} = \frac{7}{20}$$

Changing Fractions to Percentages

The easiest way to change a fraction to a percentage is to change the fraction to a decimal number first.

$$75)\overline{3.00} \;\; \frac{0.04}{} \qquad\qquad 0.04 = \frac{4}{100} = 40\%$$

Changing Percentages to Decimals

To change a percentage number to a decimal number, erase the percent sign and move the decimal point two places to the left.

$$51\% = 0.51$$

Changing Decimals to Percentages

To change the decimals numbers to percentage numbers, move the decimal point two places to the right and write in the percent sign.

$$0.76 = 76\%$$

Doing Problem With Percentages

To find a percentage of a whole number, change the percentage to a fraction or a decimal and then multiply by the whole number.

TABLE 9-2 Converting Percentages to Fractions and Decimals

Percent		Fraction		Decimal
25%	=	$\frac{1}{4}$	=	0.25
50%	=	$\frac{1}{2}$	=	0.5
75%	=	$\frac{3}{4}$	=	0.75
12.5%	=	$\frac{1}{8}$	=	0.125
37.5%	=	$\frac{3}{8}$	=	0.375
62.5%	=	$\frac{5}{8}$	=	0.625
87.5%	=	$\frac{7}{8}$	=	0.875
$33\frac{1}{3}$%	=	$\frac{1}{3}$	=	$0.33\frac{1}{3}$
$66\frac{2}{3}$%	=	$\frac{2}{3}$	=	$0.66\frac{2}{3}$
20%	=	$\frac{1}{5}$	=	0.2
40%	=	$\frac{2}{5}$	=	0.4
60%	=	$\frac{3}{5}$	=	0.6
80%	=	$\frac{4}{5}$	=	0.8
10%	=	$\frac{1}{10}$	=	0.1
30%	=	$\frac{3}{10}$	=	0.3
70%	=	$\frac{7}{10}$	=	0.7
90%	=	$\frac{9}{10}$	=	0.9
$16\frac{2}{3}$%	=	$\frac{1}{6}$	=	$0.16\frac{2}{3}$
$83\frac{1}{3}$%	=	$\frac{5}{6}$	=	$0.83\frac{1}{3}$

What is 25% of 500?

$$25\% = \frac{25}{100}$$

$$\frac{25}{100} \times 500 = 125$$

or

What is 8.5% of 250?

$$8.5\% = 0.085$$

$$0.085 \times 250 = 21.25$$

To find what percentage one number is of another number, turn the numbers in the problem into a fraction and change the fraction to a percentage.

5 is what percentage of 50?

$$\frac{5}{50} = \frac{1}{10}$$

$$\frac{1}{10} = 0.1 = 10\%$$

To find the whole number when a percentage is given, divide the whole number by the percentage. Change the percentage to a fraction.

10% of what number is 100?

$$10\% = \frac{1}{10}$$

$$100 \div \frac{1}{100} = \frac{100}{1} \times \frac{10}{1} = 1000$$

EXERCISE 9–4

Directions: Fill in the following chart. Check your work with the conversion chart in Table 9–2. Then solve problems 11 through 15.

Percent	Fraction	Decimal
1. 50%		
2.		0.125
3.	$\frac{1}{6}$	
4.		0.7
5. 60%		
6.	$\frac{2}{5}$	
7.		$0.66\frac{2}{3}$
8.	$\frac{3}{8}$	
9. 80%		
10.	$\frac{1}{4}$	

11. What is 8% of 75?
12. 18 is what percent of 16?
13. 40% of what number is 48?
14. 27 is what percent of 72?
15. 6.25% of 300 =

RATIOS

A ratio is a <u>comparison</u> of two numbers using division. A ratio can be written in three ways:

1. 16 to 32
2. $\frac{16}{32} = \frac{1}{2}$
3. 16:32

Regardless of how you write the ratio, you would read it as "16 to 32." Read the following and find out how you would solve a ratio problem.

- Of Chloe's 28 teeth, 4 have crowns on them. Determine the ratio of crowned teeth to uncrowned teeth.
- Use the 4 crowned teeth as the numerator and the total number of teeth as the denominator and reduce the fraction. $\frac{4}{28} = \frac{1}{7}$
- $\frac{1}{7}$ of Chloe's teeth are crowned.

EXERCISE 9–5

Directions: Solve the following ratio problems. Choose any of the ways to express your answer. If necessary, reduce fractions to their lowest terms.

1. At the veterinary school there are 10 instructors for 400 students. What is the ratio of instructors to students?

2. Out of 25 typed pages, the medical typist had to redo 5 of them because of errors. What is the ratio of redone pages to correct pages?

3. The laboratory assistant discovered that 6 of the 54 microscopes needed repairs. What is the ratio of working microscopes to broken ones?

4. Of the 228 graduates of the medical assistant program, 19 found jobs immediately after graduation. What is the ratio of working graduates to non-working graduates?

5. Prudence cleaned 15 of the rat cages out of a total of 50. What is the ratio of clean cages to dirty ones?

PROPORTIONS

A proportion is a statement that two ratios are equal. A proportion can be written in three ways:

1. 1 to 2 = 5 to 10
2. $\dfrac{1}{2} = \dfrac{5}{10}$
3. 1:2 = 5:10

All three of these proportions are read as "1 is to 2 as 5 is to 10." Below is what a <u>typical</u> proportion problem would look like. Determine the missing number in the following proportion:

$$\frac{?}{10} = \frac{3}{30}$$

To find the missing number, figure out what number you would multiply 10 by to get 30. The answer is 3. Earlier in this chapter you were told that whatever number you use to multiply in the denominator you must use for that numerator. So what number multiplied by 3 would equal 3? The answer is 1. The proportion equation now looks like this:

$$\frac{?}{10} = \frac{3}{30} \qquad \frac{1}{10} = \frac{3}{30}$$

EXERCISE 9–6

Directions: Write each of the following statements as a proportion.

1. 4 is to 12 as 1 is to 3.
2. 16 is to 40 as 2 is to 5.
3. 35 is to 30 as 7 is to 6.
4. 108 is to 24 as 9 is to 2.
5. 77 is to 99 as 7 is to 9.

EXERCISE 9–7

Directions: Solve the following problems by finding the value of the unknown number (?). Remember that the number that was used to determine the denominator should also be used to determine the numerator.

1. $\dfrac{4}{8} = \dfrac{?}{16}$

2. $\dfrac{5}{1} = \dfrac{35}{?}$

3. $\dfrac{45}{?} = \dfrac{5}{9}$

4. $\dfrac{?}{7} = \dfrac{18}{42}$

5. $\dfrac{7}{12} = \dfrac{?}{108}$

6. $\dfrac{40}{?} = \dfrac{4}{12}$

7. $\dfrac{18}{35} = \dfrac{108}{?}$

8. $\dfrac{51}{25} = \dfrac{?}{1000}$

9. $\dfrac{?}{76} = \dfrac{66}{228}$

10. $\dfrac{62}{909} = \dfrac{?}{1818}$

REVIEWING THE LEARNING STRATEGIES

TO LEARN	USE THIS STRATEGY
Multiplication and division	Memorize the multiplication chart
Fractions	Learn to recognize the numerator, denominator, proper and improper fractions, mixed numbers, lowest terms, and the common denominator
Decimals	Learn about place holding, reading decimal numbers, changing fractions to decimal numbers, and changing decimal numbers to fractions
Percentages	Learn about reading percentages and changing percentages to decimals or fractions
Ratios	Learn the definition of *ratio* and to read and write ratios
Proportions	Learn the definition of *proportion* and how to read and write proportions

Chapter 10

Understanding Algebra, Geometry, and the Metric System

LEARNING OBJECTIVES

In this chapter you will learn how to
- Add, subtract, multiply, and divide signed numbers
- Solve for the unknown in an equation
- Recognize four different triangles
- Find the perimeter, radius, and area of circles, squares, and rectangles
- Determine equivalent measures of the English and metric systems of measurement

VOCABULARY WORDS

The following vocabulary words are important to your understanding of the ideas in this chapter. These vocabulary words are <u>underscored</u> the first time they are used in the chapter. Read the list of words and definitions. Then check your understanding of these words before you read the chapter.

concentrate focus.

concepts ideas.

equation a mathematical expression of equality.

exponent a number written above and to the right of a number that shows how many times the number is to be multiplied by itself, for example, $4^3 = 4 \times 4 \times 4$.

extends stretches forward.

identical the same.

indicate demonstrate.

inverse opposite.

procedure steps taken in a logical manner to accomplish something.

variable a letter or symbol that represents a number of undetermined value, for example, $3x = 6$.

VOCABULARY CHECK

Directions: Choose the vocabulary word that best fits into the sentence.

1. The _____ reminded us how many times the number was multiplied by itself.

2. The arm of the octopus _____ way beyond its body.

3. The dental assistant was able to follow the dental _____ perfectly.

4. The _____ of adding is subtracting.

5. If you _____ while reading your textbook, you will do better on exams.

6. The algebraic _____ was hard to solve.

7. The student was nervous about learning all the different medical theories and _____.

8. The signs will _____ which direction to go.

9. The letter in the algebra problem represented the _____.

10. The nursing assistant students were wearing _____ uniforms.

ALGEBRA

Although many students get nervous at the mention of "algebra," they should realize that it is just a continuation of basic math skills. There are two ways that algebra differs from regular arithmetic: The first difference is that when you are working with algebra problems, letters will sometimes be substituted for numbers. Thus you may see a problem that would look like this:

$$a + b =$$

The second difference is that when doing algebra problems you will be working with negative numbers. A negative number is any number that has a value less than zero. When you do arithmetic problems, you are using only positive numbers, that is, any number that has a value greater than zero or zero. To see the difference between negative and positive numbers, refer to the following:

$$\text{-10 -9 -8 -7 -6 -5 -4 -3 -2 -1 0 +1 +2 +3 +4 +5 +6 +7 +8 +9 +10}$$

Number Line of Negative and Positive Numbers

The numbers to the left of zero are the negative numbers. To <u>indicate</u> a negative number, use a negative sign (⁻). (Do not confuse negative signs with minus signs.) The numbers on the right are the positive numbers. To indicate a positive number, use a positive sign (⁺). **If a number is unsigned, assume that it is positive.** Did you notice in the Number Line of Negative and Positive Numbers that the zero was unsigned? Zeros are neither positive nor negative. They do not require a sign.

Adding Signed Numbers

When you do algebra problems, you will add, subtract, multiply, and divide. However, since you are working with signed numbers, doing these operations will be different from what you remember doing with arithmetic. Here are the two strategies for adding signed numbers.

1. When adding numbers with signs that are the same, add and put the sign of the numbers in the answer.

$$^+3 + {}^+6 = {}^+9$$

$$^-3 + {}^-6 = {}^-9$$

2. When adding numbers with different signs, subtract and put the sign of the largest number in the answer.

$$^-8 - {^+2} = {^-6}$$
$$^+5 - {^-1} = {^+4}$$

Occasionally you will be asked to add more than two signed numbers. Here are the strategies for adding more than two numbers with mixed signs:

1. Add the numbers with positive signs.

2. Add the numbers with negative signs.

3. Subtract the two subtotals and use the sign of the largest total in your answer.

$$^-6 + {^+3} + {^-4} + {^+8}$$
$$^+3 + {^+8} = {^+11}$$
$$^-6 + {^-4} = {^-10}$$
$$^+11 + {^-10} = {^+1}$$

EXERCISE 10–1

Directions: Solve the following addition problems. Pay close attention to the signs. If they are the same in the problem, add and copy the sign into the answer. If the signs are different in the problem, subtract and copy the sign of the larger number in the answer. When adding many signed numbers, add the positive numbers first and then the negative numbers. Subtract the subtotal and copy the sign of the largest subtotal into your answer.

1. $^+4 + {^+1} =$

2. $^-5 + {^-7} =$

3. $^+6 + {^-3} =$

4. $25 + 10 =$

5. $^-66 + {^-40} =$

6. $800 + {^-245} =$

7. $^+3 + {^+7} + {^-8} + {^-1} =$

8. $^-37 + {^+86} + {^-91} + {^+10} =$

9. $^+108 + {^+22} + {^+439} + {^-151} =$

10. $^-751 + {^-488} + {^-296} + {^-300} =$

Subtracting Signed Numbers

Again, when you subtract signed numbers, the procedure is different than when you subtract in arithmetic. There are two steps for subtracting signed numbers.

1. When subtracting signed numbers, change the sign of the number being subtracted to the opposite sign.
2. Then *add* the numbers. The numbers in the following problem are in parentheses so you can clearly see the sign that will tell you what operation to do.

$$(^-9) - (^+5) =$$
$$(^-9) + (^-5) =$$
$$(^-9) + (^-5) = {}^-14$$

and

$$(^+12) - (^+2) =$$
$$(^+12) + (^-2) =$$
$$(^+12) + (^-2) = {}^+10$$

EXERCISE 10–2

Directions: Solve the following problems. Remember to change the sign of the second number to its opposite and then follow the same strategies for adding signed numbers.

1. $(^-4) - (^-1) =$
2. $(8) - (^-7) =$
3. $(^+13) - (^-13) =$
4. $(^-89) - (^-89) =$
5. $(^-751) - (232) =$
6. $(1359) - (780) =$
7. $(41,225) - (6,921) =$
8. $(^-34,109) - (29,999) =$
9. $(^+1,000,000) - (^-1,000,000) =$
10. $(^-2,000,000) - (^-1,000,000) =$

Multiplying Signed Numbers

To multiply signed numbers, you do the same as you would in arithmetic. However, to determine what sign to put in the answer, follow these two strategies:

1. If the signs in the numbers you are multiplying are the same, use the positive sign in the answer.

$$(^+25)(^+4) = {}^+100$$

2. If the signs in the numbers you are multiplying are different, use the negative sign in the answer.

$$(^{+}10)(^{-}5) = ^{-}50$$

You may have noticed in these problems that the $\times$ sign was not used to indicate multiplication. Instead, there are three ways to signal a multiplication problem in algebra.

1. The numbers will be in parentheses with no sign between them.

$$(2)(7)$$

2. A letter and a number will be next to each other.

$$3b$$

3. There will be a dot between the numbers. This way is discouraged because it could be misread as a decimal number.

$$2 \bullet 7$$

When you need to multiply more than two numbers, multiply the first two numbers and get a subtotal. Then use this subtotal to multiply with the third number.

$$(4)(2)(^{-}3)$$
$$(8)(^{-}3) = ^{-}24$$

When you are multiplying, what sign do you use for the answer? To determine the sign, *concentrate* on the negative signs. If there is an even number (2, 4, 6, etc.) of negative signs in the original problem, make the answer positive ($^{+}$). If there is an odd number (1, 3, 5, etc.) of negative signs in the problem, make the answer negative ($^{-}$). Look again, at the problem above. There were how many negative signs in the original problem? One is the answer. One is an odd number, so put a negative sign in the answer.

$$(4)(2)(^{-}3) =$$
$$(8)(^{-}3) = ^{-}24$$

and

$$(^{-}10)(^{-}2)(^{+}2) =$$
$$(20)(2) =$$
$$(20)(2) = ^{+}40$$

Count the number of negative signs in the original problem. Two is the answer. Since two is an even number, use a positive sign for the answer.

| | EXERCISE 10–3 |

Directions: Solve the following problems. Pay attention to the signs in the problem so you will know what sign to use in the answer.

1. $(4)(2) =$
2. $(^-7)(3) =$
3. $(16)(28) =$
4. $(^-135)(^-65) =$
5. $(^-202)(10) =$
6. $(^-1000)(^-88) =$
7. $(^-2)(3)(^-4) =$
8. $(10)(^-5)(2) =$
9. $(^-12)(^-3)(^+14)(^+2) =$
10. $(40)(50)(60)(^-70) =$

Dividing Signed Numbers

Dividing signed numbers is similar to multiplying signed numbers. You will need to figure out what sign to put in the answer the same way you did for the multiplication problems. If the signs in the problem are different, use the negative sign in the answer. If the signs in the problem are similar, use the positive sign in the answer.

$$^-30 \div {}^+10 = {}^-3$$
$$\frac{^-20}{^-5} = {}^+4$$

Note that the second problem is set up like a fraction. The line means "divided by." So the problem reads "$^-20$ divided by $^-5$."

| | EXERCISE 10–4 |

Directions: Solve the following problems. Pay attention to the signs so you will know what sign to use in the answer.

1. $^-2 \div {}^-6 =$
2. $^-5 \div 25 =$
3. $100 \div 1000 =$
4. $75 \div {}^-600 =$
5. $^-384 \div {}^-32 =$

6. $\dfrac{^{-}8}{^{-}4} =$

7. $\dfrac{55}{^{+}11} =$

8. $\dfrac{90}{20} =$

9. $\dfrac{150}{^{-}30} =$

10. $\dfrac{^{-}222}{^{-}111} =$

Solving Equations

As was mentioned earlier in this chapter, one of the main differences between algebra and arithmetic is that algebra uses both numbers and letters in problems. An algebraic expression that uses numbers and letters and shows how two statements are equal is called an <u>equation</u>. An equation can look like the following:

$$a + 2 = 10$$
$$m - 2 = 15$$
$$20 = 5c$$
$$\frac{9}{b} = 3$$

Working With Equations

When working with equations, it is your responsibility to find the value of the letter or, in other words, what number the letter in the equation stands for. The letter in the equation is called the "unknown" or <u>variable</u>.

- An equation is said to have two sides—a right side and a left side. The equal sign (=) separates the right and left sides.
- To solve equations, you must use <u>inverse</u> operations.
- Addition is the opposite, or inverse, of subtraction.
- Subtraction is the opposite, or inverse, of addition.
- Multiplication is the opposite, or inverse, of division.
- Division is the opposite, or inverse, of multiplication.
- To solve an equation, perform inverse operations **on both sides of the equation** until you get an answer that states "the unknown = a certain value or number."

$$? = 50$$

Using Addition in Equations

Consider the following problem:

$$x + 10 = 15$$

In this example, x is the unknown and 10 is being added to it. To find out what x stands for, do the opposite or inverse operation. The opposite operation of addition is subtraction. Subtract 10 from the left side of the equation and do the same on the right side.

$$
\begin{array}{rcr}
x + 10 = & & 15 \\
-10 & & -10 \\
\hline
0 & & 5 \\
x = 5 &
\end{array}
$$

You know you have solved the equation when the variable is on one side of the equal sign and a number is on the other.

Using Subtraction in Equations

Look at the next example.

$$20 = b - 8$$

You notice that in this problem 8 is being subtracted from b. To solve this equation and find the value of b, do the opposite or inverse operation to both sides of the equation. Addition is the inverse of subtraction.

$$
\begin{array}{l}
20 = b - 8 \\
b = 20 + 8 \\
28 = b
\end{array}
$$

Keep in mind the strategy for adding signed numbers. Look at the right side of the equation. When adding unlike signs, subtract and keep the sign of the larger number. The 8s, however, cancel out each other. On the left side, the signs are the same. Add the 20 and the 8; the answer is $28 = b$.

Using Multiplication in Equations

Study the following problem:

$$11s = 33$$

Because this is a multiplication problem, you need to do the inverse operation, which is division. Divide both sides of the equation by 11.

$$\frac{11}{11s} = \frac{33}{11}$$

$$1s = 3s = 3$$

On the left side of this problem, you divide 11 by 11. The answer, of course, is 1. It is not necessary to write 1 in algebra because the variable stands for 1 automatically.

Remember that your aim in solving equations is having the unknown or variable on one side of the equal sign and a number value on the other side.

Using Division in Equations

Think about this final equation problem.

$$\frac{p}{5}=15$$

To solve this problem, you will have to do the inverse operation for division. You will have to multiply by 5 on both sides of the equal sign. The example should look like this:

$$\frac{p}{5}=15$$

$$(5)\ \frac{p}{5}=15$$

$$p = 75$$

Remember that when you do any inverse multiplication or division on <u>identical</u> numbers, the result will always be one; when you use inverse addition and subtraction on identical numbers, the result will always be zero.

Checking Your Answer

The method for checking your answer when solving an equation is simple. Regardless of the operation you did, substitute the number you arrived at for the unknown in the problem. Consider the last problem.

$$\frac{p}{5}=15$$

Substitute the 75 you have for your answer for p.

$$\frac{75}{5} = 15$$

If the equation is true, you know that you have the right solution.

EXERCISE 10–5

Directions: Solve and check the following equations. Pay attention to what operations you need to do to get the correct answers.

1. $c + 14 = 30$
2. $9 = p + 3$
3. $k - 13 = 3$
4. $25 = m - 5$
5. $36k = 9$

6. $100 = 10v$

7. $\dfrac{b}{88} = 11$

8. $64 = \dfrac{k}{7}$

9. $372 = 12n$

10. $\dfrac{x}{5} = 1$

GEOMETRY

Geometry is the part of mathematics that deals with the measuring of lines, angles, and shapes. As long as you are familiar with certain geometric terms and <u>concepts</u> you should have no trouble doing geometry problems.

Basic Geometry Terms

- A **point** is a precise location in space. Because it cannot be seen, a dot (·) is used to represent a point.

- A **line** is an endless set of points. In geometry, a line with an arrow at each end represents a line.

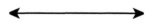

- An **angle** is formed when two straight lines meet at one point. Angles are measured in degrees from 0° to 360°.

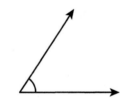

In geometry the common shapes are

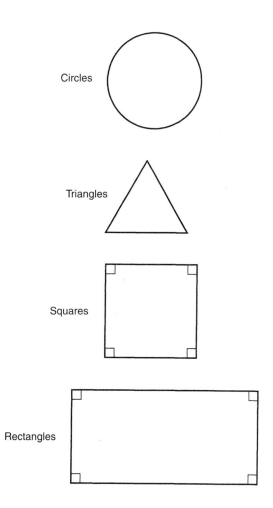

Circles

Triangles

Squares

Rectangles

Circles

A circle is a round shape with points that are an equal distance from the center. The **radius** (*r*) of the circle is a line that starts at the center and <u>extends</u> to the circle.

The **diameter** (*d*) is a line that starts at the circle, goes through the radius, and ends at the opposite side of the circle.

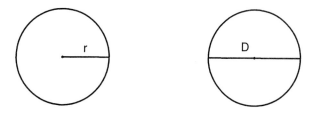

Finding the Diameter of a Circle

The diameter of a circle is twice as long as the radius. Therefore, to find the diameter of a circle, you multiply the radius by 2. Consider the following problem:

What is the diameter of a circle with a 10-inch radius? First, write the formula for finding the diameter. Note that d stands for diameter, r stands for the radius, and (2) means that you multiply the radius by 2.

$$d = r(2)$$

Next substitute a number for its letter. Place 10 in the problem for r.

$$d = 10(2)$$

Complete the problem. Multiply 10 by 2.

$$d = 20$$

The answer is 20 inches.

Finding the Radius of a Circle

To find the radius of a circle when the diameter is given, simply divide the diameter by 2.

$$r = d \div 2$$

Follow the steps for the next problem:

What is the radius of a circle with a diameter of 10 inches?

Since the radius of a circle is half the size of the diameter, divide the diameter by 2.

$$10 \div 2 = 5$$

The answer is 5 inches.

Finding the Circumference of a Circle

The circumference (c) of a circle is the measurement of the distance around the entire circle.

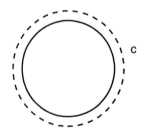

When trying to determine the relationship of the circumference to the diameter of any circle, you must do a ratio (*c/d*). However, when you use actual numbers to determine the ratio, you will create a nonending decimal. To simplify this fraction, the pi symbol is used (π). The value of pi is approximately 3.14, making the nonending decimal much more manageable.

Determining the Area of a Circle

The area (*a*) of a circle is all the space within the circle. To determine the area of a circle, you must understand a simple formula:

$$a = (\pi)r^2$$

In this formula, *a* = area; (π) = pi or 3.14; r^2 = radius multiplied by itself.
Look at the following problem:
If a circle has a radius 10 inches, what is the area?
To solve this problem, you must remove the letters and substitute the numbers given in the problem.

$$a = \pi r^2$$
$$a = 3.14 \,(10 \times 10)$$

Then work the numbers in parenthesis first. The r^2 means that you multiply a number by its own value. In other words, multiply the radius of 10 by 10.

$$10 \times 10 = 100$$

Then multiply the answer by the value of pi.

$$3.14(100) = 314 \text{ inches.}$$

The area of the circle is 314 square inches.

EXERCISE 10–6

Directions: Solve the following problems.

1. What is the radius of a circle with a 20-inch diameter?

2. What is the radius of a circle with a 1-inch diameter?

3. What is the radius of a circle with a $9\frac{1}{2}$ inch diameter?

4. What is the diameter of a circle with a 7-inch radius?

5. What is the diameter of a circle with a 25-inch radius?

6. What is the diameter of a circle with a $\frac{3}{4}$-inch radius?

7. What is the area of a circle with a 5-inch radius?

8. What is the area of a circle with an 11-inch radius?

9. What is the area of a circle with a 25-inch radius?

10. What is the area of a circle with a $\frac{1}{10}$-inch radius?

Triangles

Triangle means "three angles," so all triangles contain three inside angles. These angles are measured in degrees (°). When you add up the number of degrees in a triangle, **it always equals 180° degrees.**

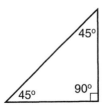

Types of Triangles

An **equilateral** triangle, as its name suggests, has three sides of equal length. Because the three sides are of equal length, the three angles are also equal. In other words, the three angles, which are measured in degrees, consist of the same number of degrees. Since the sum of all angles in a triangle equals 180 degrees, each of the three angles in an equilateral triangle is 180° ÷ 3 = 60°.

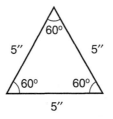

An **isosceles** triangle has two sides of equal length. The angles opposite the equal sides are equal also.

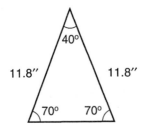

A **right** triangle has an angle that measures 90°. This creates one side that is longer than the other two sides. This side opposite the right angle is called the **hypotenuse**.

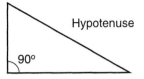

Depending on how it is drawn, an isosceles triangle can also be a right triangle. A **scalene** triangle has no sides that are equal. The angles are unequal also.

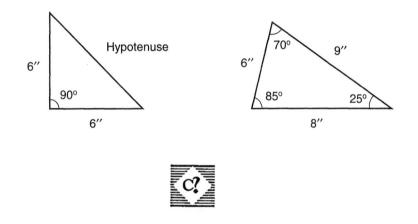

EXERCISE 10-7

Directions: Below is a chart representing three types of triangles—equilateral, isosceles, and scalene. Fill in the chart. Remember that the sum of all angles must equal 180°. The first has been done for you.

Types of Triangle	Angle *A*	Angle *B*	Angle *C*
equilateral	60	60	60
scalene	23	55	
right (isosceles)		45	
	35.5		35.5
	18.2	66	95.8
isosceles	15		
	99.4	3.6	
right			
scalene			
isosceles			

Squares

A square is a shape with four equal sides. The four angles are equal also. The angles of a square are right angles and equal 360°.

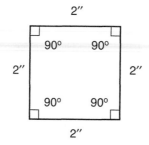

Finding the Perimeter of a Square

The **perimeter** of a square is the entire distance around the edges of the square. You can find the perimeter in two ways. The first way is to measure one side and, since all the sides are equal, add up the lengths of all four sides. The formula for finding the perimeter in this way is:

$$p = s1 + s2 + s3 + s4$$
$$8 = 2 + 2 + 2 + 2$$

In this formula, p stands for perimeter and s for side. The second way of determing the perimeter of a square is to measure one side and then multiply by 4. The formula looks like this:

$$p = 4s$$
$$48 = (4)(12)$$

EXERCISE 10–8

Directions: Find the perimeter for each of the following problems. Use either the addition formula or the multiplication formula.

What is the perimeter of a square that measures:

1. 5 inches?

2. 10.5 inches?

3. $9\frac{1}{4}$ feet?

4. $12\frac{3}{4}$ miles?

5. 100 kilometers?

Finding the Area of a Square

The **area** of a square is how much space is in the inside of the shape. To find the area of a square, measure one side and multiply the number by itself. The formula for finding the area of a square looks like the following where the small 2 is called an <u>exponent</u> and means to "square the number" or multiply it by itself:

$$a = s^2$$
$$a = 3(3) = 9 \text{ square units}$$

(Note that the answer will also be squared.)

EXERCISE 10–9

Directions: Study the above formula for finding the area of a square. Then solve the following problems:

What is the area of a square that measures:

1. 7 inches?

2. 64 feet?

3. $4\frac{1}{2}$ miles?

4. 6,000 kilometers?

5. 2,800 yards?

Rectangles

A rectangle is a shape whose opposite sides are equal in length with all right angles. The shorter sides of a rectangle are the width and the longer sides are the length.

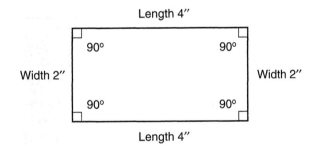

Finding the Perimeter of a Rectangle

To find the perimeter of a rectangle, add up the measurement of all four sides. Remember each side that is opposite will have the same measurement. The formula for finding the perimeter of a rectangle is:

$$p = s1 + s2 + s3 + s4$$
$$p = 2 + 4 + 2 + 4$$
$$p = 12$$

EXERCISE 10–10

Directions: Solve the following perimeter problems:
What is the perimeter of a rectangle with the following measurements?

1. width = 5; length = 8
2. width = 12 inches; length = $1\frac{1}{2}$ feet
3. width = $7\frac{1}{4}$ yards; length = $9\frac{3}{4}$ yards
4. width = 16 kilometers; length = 50 kilometers
5. width = 92 centimeters; length = 186 centimeters

Finding the Area of a Rectangle

To find the area of a rectangle, multiply length by width. The formula for determining the area of a rectangle looks like the following:

$$a = (l)(w)$$
$$a = 4 \times 2$$
$$a = 8$$

EXERCISE 10–11

Directions: Find the area for the following rectangles. Refer to the formula above if necessary.

1. length = 10, width = 4
2. length = 9.5 inches; width = 0.5 inch
3. length = $4\frac{1}{6}$ feet; width = 3 feet
4. length = 21 centimeters; width = 18 centimeters
5. length = 24 miles; width = $\frac{1}{2}$ mile

THE METRIC SYSTEM

The metric system is a system of measurements. Another system of measurements is called the English system. The United States is one of the very few countries that uses the English system of measuring. Most of the world, including the health fields, use the metric system of measuring. Therefore, it is very important to be familiar with the metric system. Table 10–1 shows how measurements in the English system and the metric system are equivalent. Since some of the equivalent numbers can be long and complicated decimal numbers, they have been rounded off.

TABLE 10–1   Metric System and English System Conversion Chart

Metric Lengths	English Length
1 meter =	39.37 inches
1 meter =	3.28 feet
1 meter =	1.09 yards
1 centimeter =	0.4 inch
1 millimeter =	0.04 inch
1 kilometer =	0.62 mile
English Lengths	**Metric Lengths**
1 inch =	25.4 millimeters
1 inch =	2.54 centimeters
1 inch =	0.0254 meter
1 foot =	0.3 meter
1 yard =	0.91 meter
1 mile =	1.61 kilometers
Metric Liquid Measures	**English Liquid Measures**
1 liter =	1.06 quarts
English Liquid Measures	**Metric Liquid Measures**
1 quart =	0.95 liter
Metric Measure Of Weight	**English Measure Of Weight**
1 gram =	0.04 ounce
1 kilogram =	2.2 pounds
1 metric ton =	2204.62 pounds
English Measure Of Weight	**Metric Measure Of Weight**
1 ounce =	28.35 grams
1 pound =	0.45 kilogram
1 short ton (2000 pounds) =	0.91 metric ton
Metric Measure Of Area	**English Measure Of Area**
1 square centimeter =	0.155 square inch
1 square meter =	10.76 square feet
1 square meter=	1.2 square yards
1 square kilometer =	0.39 square mile
English Measure Of Area	**Metric Measure Of Area**
1 square inch =	6.45 square centimeters
1 square foot =	0.09 square meter
1 square yard =	0.84 square meter
1 square mile =	2.59 square kilometers

To change from the metric system to the English system, multiply the amount of the metric measure by its equivalent in the English system. For example, to change 5 kilometers to miles, multiply 5 kilometers by 0.62 miles.

$$5 \times 0.62 = 3.1 \text{ miles}$$

To change from the English system to the metric system, multiply the amount of the English measure by its equivalent in the metric system. For example, to change 2 inches to centimeters, multiply 2 inches by 2.54 centimeters.

$$2 \times 2.54 = 5.08 \text{ centimeters}$$

EXERCISE 10–12

Directions: Study Table 10–1. Then answer the following questions.
Change the following liters to quarts:

1. 3 liters
2. 18 liters

Change the following square centimeters to square inches:

3. 9 square centimeters
4. 10 square centimeters

Change the following kilometers to miles:

5. 4 kilometers
6. 30 kilometers

Change the following yards to meters:

7. 7 yards
8. 45 yards

Change the following pounds to kilograms:

9. 18 pounds
10. 50 pounds

REVIEWING THE LEARNING STRATEGIES

TO LEARN	**USE THIS STRATEGY**
Addition of signed numbers with the same sign	Add and use that sign in the answer
Addition of signed numbers with different signs	Subtract and use the sign of the larger number in the answer
Subtraction of signed numbers	Change the sign of the number being subtracted and add
Multiplication of signed numbers	If signs are similar, the product is positive If signs are different, the product is negative
Division of signed numbers	If signs are the same, the quotient is positive If signs are different, the quotient is negative
To solve for the unknown in an equation	Use inverse operations
To find the diameter of a circle	$d = r(2)$
To find the radius of a circle when the diameter is given	$r = d \div 2$
To find the area of a circle	$a = \pi r^2$
About triangles	Review the definitions of equilateral, isosceles, right, and scalene triangles
To find the perimeter of a square	$p = s1 + s2 + s3 + s4,\ p = 4s$
To find the area of a square	$a = s^2$
To find the perimeter of a rectangle	$p = s1 + s2 + s3 + s4$
To find the area of a rectangle	$a = (l)(w)$
To convert from the English system to the metric system or from the metric system to the English system	Review the equivalent chart

Chapter
11

Solving Word Problems

LEARNING OBJECTIVES

In this chapter you will learn how to
- Carefully read word problems
- Clarify the information in word problems
- Determine the correct operations to use for solving word problems
- Check your answer

VOCABULARY WORDS

The following vocabulary words are important to your understanding of the ideas in this chapter. These vocabulary words are underscored the first time they are used in the chapter. Read the list of words and definitions. Then check your understanding of these words before you read the chapter.

data factual information, usually in number form.

formulate devise.

intimidated made timid or fearful.

logically relating to the ability to use reason.

product the answer in a multiplication problem.

quadrupled made four times greater.

quantity amount or total.

quotient the answer in a division problem.

respectively in the given order.

sum the answer in an addition problem.

VOCABULARY CHECK

Directions: Choose the vocabulary word that best fits into the sentence.

1. He _____ his money by investing wisely.

2. You purchased the right amount; the _____ was perfect.

3. Three is the _____ of 6 divided by 2.

4. He keyed in all the statistical _____ on his computer.

5. The bully _____ the young school child.

6. The _____ of 5 times 5 is 25.

7. The dime and the quarter belonged to Lulu and Mrs. Scheer, _____.

8. Eight is the _____ of 6 plus 2.

9. He worked at the puzzle very _____.

10. They will _____ the complete study schedule.

Example 11–1

Word Problem: The medical secretary typed two reports of 18 pages each. The next day she typed four reports of 21 pages, 11 pages, 16 pages, and 4 pages, <u>respectively</u>. How many times did the medical secretary go to the bubbler?

To many otherwise capable students, all word problems make as much sense as the one above. They are <u>intimidated</u> just by the idea of having to solve even the simplest word problem. The good news is that this does not have to be the case. Once you learn how to read a word problem, <u>formulate</u> your own questions and look for the signal words that will tell you what operation to perform, word problems will no longer seem as confusing as the one above.

CAREFUL READING

The first strategy to use for solving a word problem is to read the problem very carefully. This means that you have to slow down your rate of reading. If there are any words you do not understand, you should look up their meanings in a dictionary if you can. Careful reading of a word problem also means that you may have to read the problem more than once. Remember that there will be no correct solution to the word problem if you do not understand what you are reading and what the words mean.

EXERCISE 11–1

Directions: Below is an example of a word problem. Read the problem carefully. In the space provided, write the strategies you used to make the problem more understandable. Then solve the problem if you can.

Dr. Williams asked his medical secretary to check the electric and gas bills for the office. The reading for last month's electrical meter was 4,295 kilowatt hours, and this month's reading of the electric meter was 5,229 kilowatt hours. How many kilowatt hours were used in Dr. William's office this month? The medical secretary then read the gas meter and remembered that last month's reading was 6,879 hundred cubic feet and that this month's reading was 8,432 hundred cubic feet. How many hundred cubic feet of gas was used this month?

Strategies used to understand this problem: _____

_____

_____

_____

_____

Solutions to this problem: _____

FORMULATING QUESTIONS

Once you feel that you understand the problem, the second strategy for solving word problems is to formulate or create questions to help you begin to solve the problem. The types of questions you can use to aid you in answering the word problems are as follows:

1. What <u>data</u> or numbers are given in the problem?
   Make a list of all the numbers from the word problem on a separate piece of paper. The numbers in a word problem are the heart of the problem. Make sure you are seeing them correctly by rewriting them.
2. What is the question being asked?
   It is important that you recognize the sentence that is asking you to perform a specific mathematical operation. This is a major step in solving the word problem. Table 11–1 lists some of the words used for the question sentence in a word problem.

TABLE 11–1   Some Words Used in the Question Sentence of a Word Problem

Question Word	Example
How	How many are there?
	How much does it cost?
What	What is the total?
Where	Where are the most trees?
When	When will he return?
Which	Which brother is older?
	Which is more expensive?
Who	Who spent the most money?

3. What operation do you use?

    There are words in the problem that will tell you how to solve the word problem. These specific signal words will be discussed later in the chapter.

4. Does my answer make sense?

    This is the question you will use to prove that your answer is correct. In a word problem, you need to check to see whether your answer <u>logically</u> relates to the other numbers in the problem. In other words, you need to determine whether your answer is too large or too small on the basis of the data supplied.

EXERCISE 11–2

Directions: Read the following word problem. Then answer the questions in the space provided.

Serena is reading her physics book. She learns that the speed of sound is 1,088 feet per second. She also learns that the speed of light is 186,324 miles per second. How far does sound travel in 2 hours? How far does light travel in 2 hours?

1. What are the data in the problem? List these numbers.

    _____

    _____

    _____

2. What are the questions being asked?

    _____

    _____

    _____

    _____

3. What are the answers to this problem? (Hint: In the problem you were given the length of time in **seconds**. Since you are being asked for the length of time in

hours, a greater measure of time, you multiply. Also, there are 3,600 seconds in 1 hour.)

_____

_____

4. Does my answer make sense in relation to the numbers in the problem?

_____

_____

SIGNAL WORDS

As mentioned earlier in this chapter, there are signal words that will tell you what operation to do to solve the word problem. Once you learn to recognize these signal words, you will be able to answer most word problems. The signal words will help you recognize addition, subtraction, multiplication, and division word problems.

Signal Words in Addition Problems

If you see the words in Table 11–2 in a word problem, use addition to get the answer.

EXERCISE 11–3

Directions: Read the following word problems. Answer the questions in the space provided.

A. There are three laboratories in the veterinary school. The first lab has 6 Bunsen burners; the second lab has 5 Bunsen burners and the third lab has 11 Bunsen burners. How many Bunsen burners are in the veterinary school all together?

1. What are the data in this problem?

_____

_____

TABLE 11–2   Addition Signal Words

Addition Word	Example
Add	Add the 2 totals together.
Added to	5 was added to 2.
All together	How much was spent all together?
Both	How far did both kids run?
How much	How much did the 3 cats cost?
In all	How many chickens in all were sold?
Increased by	Her waist increased by how many inches?
More than	Peppy has 2 more books than Leslie's 4 books.
Plus	5 rugs plus 4 rugs equal how many rugs?
Sum	The sum of 18 and 19 is what?
Total	What is the total number of fat rats?

2. What question is asked in the problem?

_____

_____

_____

3. What is the question word or words?

_____

_____

4. What are the signal words?

_____

5. What operation do you do to get the answer?

_____

6. What is the answer to the word problem?

_____

7. Does your answer make sense in relation to the numbers in the problem?

_____

B. Three hundred twenty-two persons applied to the dental school in Chicago. Four hundred three persons applied to the dental school in Boston. Six hundred fifty-nine persons applied to the dental school in Atlanta. What is the total number of persons applying to dental schools in Chicago, Boston, and Atlanta?

1. What are the data in this problem?

_____

_____

2. What question is asked in the problem?

_____

_____

_____

3. What is the question word or words?

_____

_____

4. What are the signal words?

_____

5. What operation do you do to get the answer?

_____

6. What is the answer to the word problem?

_____

7. Does your answer make sense in relation to the numbers in the problem?

_____

Signal Words in Subtraction Problems

If you see the words in Table 11–3 in a word problem, use subtraction to get the answer.

EXERCISE 11–4

Directions: Read the following word problems. Answer the questions in the space provided.

A. Mr. Francis is 5 feet 8 inches tall. Mrs. Francis is smaller than Mr. Francis by 4 inches. How tall is Mrs. Francis?

1. What are the data in this problem?

_____

_____

2. What question is asked in the problem?

_____

_____

_____

3. What is the question word or words?

_____

_____

4. What are the signal words?

_____

5. What operation do you do to get the answer?

_____

TABLE 11–3   Subtraction Signal Words

Subtraction Words	Example
Decreased by	His allowance was decreased by $2.
Difference	What was the difference in salary?
Fewer	How many fewer dogs are there?
Have left	How many eggs does she have left?
Left over	How much dough was left over?
Less than	He has 6 boats less than his brother.
Remain	17 cups remain out of 20.
Smaller than	Gabrielle is smaller by 6 inches than Josephina.
Subtract	Subtract 10 from 100.
Take away	11 take away 2 equals what?

6. What is the answer to the word problem?

   _____

7. Does your answer make sense in relation to the numbers in the problem?

   _____

B. Benny's studying time has been decreased by 8 hours. Before this, he was able to study 24 hours per week. How many study hours remain for Benny?

   1. What are the data in this problem?

      _____

      _____

   2. What question is asked in the problem?

      _____

      _____

      _____

   3. What is the question word or words?

      _____

      _____

   4. What are the signal words?

      _____

   5. What operation do you do to get the answer?

      _____

6. What is the answer to the word problem?

_____

7. Does your answer make sense in relation to the numbers in the problem?

_____

Signal Words in Multiplication Problems

If you see the words in Table 11–4 in a word problem, use multiplication to get the answer.

In addition to these signal words, you may see an occasional word problem that will tell you the <u>quantity</u> of one item and ask you to find the quantity of many items. For example, the problem will give you the price or length of an object and will ask you to find the price or length of 10 objects. Multiply when you see this kind of problem.

EXERCISE 11–5

Directions: Read the following word problems. Answer the questions in the space provided.

A. Jon's rate of reading is 250 words per minute. How many words can he read in an hour?

1. What are the data in this problem?

_____

_____

2. What question is asked in the problem?

_____

_____

_____

3. What is the question word or words?

_____

_____

4. What are the signal words?

_____

5. What operation do you do to get the answer?

_____

TABLE 11–4   Multiplication Signal Words

Multiplication Words	Example
Double, triple, etc.	Recently, his salary doubled.
Multiply	Multiply $5 by 4 weeks.
Product (answer in a multiplication problem)	What is the product of 94 multiplied by 6?
Times	What does 9 times 2 equal?

6. What is the answer to the word problem?

7. Does your answer make sense in relation to the numbers in the problem?

B. Carole earned $1000 per week last year. This year she received a raise that quadrupled her salary. How much is she earning now?

1. What are the data in this problem?

2. What question is asked in the problem?

3. What is the question word or words?

4. What are the signal words?

5. What operation do you do to get the answer?

6. What is the answer to the word problem?

7. Does your answer make sense in relation to the numbers in the problem?

Signal Words in Division Problems

If you see the words in Table 11–5 in a word problem, use division to get the answer.

In addition to these signal words, you may see a word problem that tells you the value of many items and asks you to figure out the value of one item. For example, the problem will give you the width or size of many objects and will ask you to figure out the width or size of one object. Use division when you see this kind of problem.

EXERCISE 11–6

Directions: Read the following word problems. Answer the questions in the space provided.

A. Melissa is 9 years 10 months old. Her younger sister Lauren is half of that age. How old is Lauren?

1. What are the data in this problem?

   _____

   _____

2. What question is asked in the problem?

   _____

   _____

   _____

3. What is the question word or words?

   _____

   _____

4. What are the signal words?

   _____

5. What operation do you do to get the answer?

   _____

TABLE 11–5   Division Signal Words

Division Words	Example
Divide	Divide the cost of the car by 12 months.
Half of	Half of 900 is what?
Separate	Separate the 12 apples into 6 containers.
Quotient (answer in a division problem)	What is the quotient of 81 divided by 9?

6. What is the answer to the word problem?

_____

7. Does your answer make sense in relation to the numbers in the problem?

_____

B. Video tapes were on sale. The cost for 12 videos was $250.00. What was the cost of 1 video?

1. What are the data in this problem?

_____

_____

2. What question is asked in the problem?

_____

_____

3. What is the question word or words?

_____

_____

4. What are the signal words?

_____

5. What operation do you do to get the answer?

_____

6. What is the answer to the word problem?

_____

7. Does your answer make sense in relation to the numbers in the problem?

_____

PRACTICING WHAT YOU HAVE LEARNED

EXERCISE 11–7

Directions: Following are some word problems. Read the problems carefully to make sure you understand what you need to do to correctly answer the questions. On a separate piece of paper, make up your own questions or answer the questions above to clarify the problems further. Look for the question and signal words that will tell you what operations you need to do to answer the questions. Write the answers in the space provided.

1. The LPN was responsible for carrying 5 trays of food on Sunday, 7 trays on Monday, 9 trays on Tuesday, 11 trays on Wednesday, 5 trays again on Thursday, 6 on Friday, and none on Saturday. What is the total number of trays the LPN carried in a week?

   Answer _____

2. How many trays of food did the LPN carry in 13 weeks?

   Answer _____

3. The radiographic technician earns $36,000 per year. What is his monthly salary?

   Answer _____

4. The health care student bought her uniform on sale. The original price was $32.98. The store was willing to reduce the price $2.95. How much does the student have to spend to buy the uniform?

   Answer _____

5. Larry wants to buy a medical dictionary that costs $75.00. He is able to pay half in cash and the rest in equal payments for 6 months. How much are Larry's monthly payments?

   Answer _____

6. Elizabeth is the smartest student in her dental hygienist program. She studies $4\frac{1}{4}$ hourson Monday, $2\frac{1}{2}$ hours on Tuesday, and $8\frac{3}{4}$ hours on both Saturday and Sunday. How many hours does Elizabeth study per week?

   Answer _____

7. There are 245 women in the medical assistant's program and 5 men. What percentage of the class is male?

   Answer _____

8. Tony works in the lab for $8\frac{1}{2}$ hours every day for a week. What is the total number of hours Tony works in the lab?

   Answer _____

9. Mr. Roth made $9\frac{1}{8}$ quarts of the solution. He wants to keep the solution in flasks that hold $1\frac{1}{2}$ quarts each. How many flasks will he need?

Answer _____

10. The mileage on the ambulance reads 32,980.7 miles. The ambulance is driven 1,003.2 miles more. What is the new mileage?

Answer _____

11. Lisa runs the 40-yard long hospital corridor in 13.8 seconds. Tom runs the same corridor in 15.9 seconds. How much slower is Tom?

Answer _____

12. The bus fare to the medical center was raised from $1.00 to $1.25. A student needs to take the bus twice a day, Monday through Friday. How much more will the student spend on bus fare per week?

Answer _____

13. The cost of 10 cans of soda pop in the hospital cafeteria is $7.70 What is the cost of 1 can of pop?

Answer _____

14. Blossom typed $\frac{1}{8}$ of the medical report on Monday. She typed $\frac{1}{4}$ of the medical report on Tuesday. How much of the medical report does Blossom need to type to finish it on Wednesday?

Answer _____

15. Michael uses $2\frac{3}{4}$ ounces of alcohol in a solution. How many ounces of alcohol does he need to make $\frac{1}{4}$ of the solution?

Answer _____

16. Sara cut gauze that was $1\frac{1}{3}$ yards long into four bandages. How long was each bandage?

Answer _____

17. The phlebotomy program has 700 students this year. The program's assistant director must order 95 syringes for each of the students. What is the product of 700 times 95?

Answer _____

18. The head of the dental assistant's program makes $60,000 annually. The financial officer of the program wants to know how much the head of the program makes monthly. What is the quotient of $60,000 divided by 12?

    Answer _____

19. You were assigned 225 pages to read. You finished $\frac{1}{4}$ of them. How many pages remain to be read?

    Answer _____

20. Dr. T. Brown collected $2,265 in patients' fees for one day. He saw 30 patients that day. How much money did each patient pay to the doctor?

    Answer _____

REVIEWING THE LEARNING STRATEGIES

TO LEARN	USE THIS STRATEGY
To read word problems carefully	Slow down reading rate
	Look up unknown words in the dictionary
	Reread problem
To clarify word problems	Answer these questions:
	What are the data given?
	What is the question being asked?
To determine what mathematical operation to do	Learn signal words for addition, subtraction, multiplication, and division.
To check your answer	Answer this question: Does my answer make sense in relation to the data given in the problem?

UNIT IV

STUDY STRATEGIES

Learning study strategies will help you organize your time and information so that you will become a more efficient learner. You will find that applying these strategies to the subjects you are studying will give you a plan to keep up with your assignments and achieve better grades. Chapter 12, Managing Time, will teach you how to set and prioritize goals, schedule your study time, and eliminate distractions. Chapter 13, Learning Active Listening Skills, will demonstrate how applying active listening strategies will help you to improve your concentration during lectures. Chapter 14, Taking Notes, will give you the strategies you need to focus on the important information in your lectures and textbooks. Chapter 15, Improving Test Scores, will teach you five strategies to help you prepare for and take tests more successfully. Applying the study strategies discussed in this unit will help you to improve your work habits and your test results.

Chapter
12

Managing Time

LEARNING OBJECTIVE

In this chapter you will learn how to
• Organize your time so that you will improve your study habits.

VOCABULARY WORDS

The following vocabulary words are important to your understanding of the ideas in this chapter. These vocabulary words are underscored the first time they are used in the chapter. Read the list of words and definitions. Then check your understanding of these words before you read the chapter.

academic having to do with school or learning.
anxiety emotional pain.
external outside the body.
goals aims, intentions.
internal inside the body.
juggling dealing with several things at one time.
prioritize in order of importance.
procrastination delaying what needs to be done.
recreational having to do with activities designed for relaxation and fun.
tendency leaning toward.

VOCABULARY CHECK

Directions: Choose the vocabulary word that best fits into the sentence.

1. Cynthia was filled with _____ because she was unprepared for her chemistry exam.

2. Tennis is a popular _____ activity.

3. Please _____ your concerns so that we can take care of them in order of importance.

4. _____ home and work responsibilities is often difficult.

5. Tarry has a _____ to manipulate a situation.

6. Maria worked hard to reach all her _____.

7. Jeffrey's habit of _____ prevents him from finishing his assignments on time.

8. _____ events such as work pressures intruded on her personal life.

9. _____ thoughts kept Robert from concentrating on what the speaker was announcing.

10. The school offers a wide range of _____ subjects because it has a varied curriculum.

HOW TO MANAGE TIME

Many students find that they have difficulty getting started on assignments. As the semester goes on, they suddenly realize that they have fallen so far behind that it is difficult to catch up. Learning strategies for managing time will help you to avoid that problem. You will learn how to organize your time by

- Setting goals
- Learning to <u>prioritize</u>

- Scheduling
- Eliminating distractions
- Monitoring your ability to manage time
- Avoiding <u>procrastination</u>

SETTING GOALS

Establish <u>goals</u> for the semester as a whole. What do you want to accomplish by the end of the semester? When setting semester goals, you have to think about all your responsibilities and interests. How many courses are you planning to take during the semester?

Are you working while attending school? Do you work part-time or full-time? Day or evening? What are your home and family responsibilities? Do you have special hobbies, <u>recreational</u> interests, or volunteer activities?

Sometimes you can feel overwhelmed by all that you need to do. A solution is to make a list of your goals like the one that follows. List everything you want to achieve for the semester. Make sure that your goals are balanced. Allow some recreational time. It is not realistic to plan your semester with just study and work.

One Student's Semester Goals

- Taking full-time schedule at school to become a dental hygienist
- Practice piano 5 hours a week
- Grocery shopping for family
- Volunteer tutoring at public library 1 hour a week
- Part-time job 8 hours a week

EXERCISE 12–1

Directions: Make a list of your semester goals

_____

_____

_____

_____

_____

PRIORITIZING GOALS

Prioritizing goals is placing your goals in order of importance to you. Think about your list of semester goals. Some are more urgent than others. When you are in school, studying for an exam should take priority over going to the movies. Keep in mind that prioritizing will help you to accomplish your most important goals first. Be realistic about what you expect to accomplish in a semester. Decide what goals are most important and focus on achieving those goals.

One Student's Prioritized Semester Goals

1. Taking full-time schedule at school to become a dental hygienist
2. Grocery shopping for family
3. Working part-time 8 hours a week
4. Practice piano 5 hours a week
5. Volunteer tutoring at public library 1 hour a week

EXERCISE 12–2

Directions: Decide what is most important to you and prioritize your list of semester goals.

_____

_____

_____

_____

_____

SCHEDULING

Planning and following a schedule will help you to organize your time. Once you have decided and prioritized your semester goals, you should schedule your time so that you can realistically meet your goals. Using calendars helps you stick to a schedule. Monthly, weekly, and daily calendars will help you plan your time efficiently.

Monthly Calendar

Use monthly calendars to plan long-range assignments. Some helpful information to place on your monthly calendar:

- Test dates
- Vacation dates
- Due dates of reports and projects

EXERCISE 12–3

Directions: Fill in the monthly calendar (Fig. 12–1). List any important test dates or long-range plans on the calendar.

JANUARY

SUN	MON	TUE	WED	THURS	FRI	SAT
	1	2	3	4	5	6
7	8	9	10	11 *conference*	12	13
14	15	16	17	18 *computer applications exam*	19	20
21	22	23	24	25	26 *biology lab report due*	27
28	29	30	31			

FIGURE 12–1 A monthly calendar with special assignment dates marked.

Weekly Calendar

Using a weekly calendar will help you to organize your time and to follow a regular schedule. Successful students use weekly calendars to help them work on their assignments at scheduled times. They establish a place to study and a time to study and they follow a regular study plan.

You use a weekly calendar to organize all your activities for the week. You plan your activities at the beginning of each week and follow the schedule as closely as possible. Some of the activities you would put on your weekly schedule are class hours, work hours, mealtimes, sleep time, extracurricular activities, sports practice. Then circle the hours that are free for study. Be realistic. Allow some unscheduled time for relaxing and recreation. Once you have decided *when* you want to study, then you should decide *where* you want to study. Your choice of study place should be quiet, well lit, and free from distractions. Study wherever you will concentrate best, whether it is at home or the library. After you have decided when and where you want to study, you are beginning to get organized. Sticking to the schedule you have planned will help you to manage your time.

EXERCISE 12–4

Directions: Fill in the weekly calendar (Fig. 12–2) at the beginning of the week. As you go through the week, make a check mark next to each task you complete. You will then see at a glance whether you are accomplishing your goals. Remember, you may have to make changes in your calendar as the week progresses, but by planning your week you are learning to manage your time efficiently.

TIME	SUN	MON	TUES	WED	THURS	FRI	SAT
7–8 AM							
8–9							
9–10							
10–11							
11–12							
12–1 PM							
1–2							
2–3							
3–4							
4–5							
5–6							
6–7							
7–8							
8–9							

FIGURE 12–2 A weekly calendar.

Daily Calendar

Use the daily calendar (Fig. 12–3) to help you focus on your priorities. Each night, think about what you want to accomplish the next day. Write a "to-do" list.

To-Do List

A to-do list is your list of everything you want to accomplish the next day. The list includes both <u>academic</u> and nonacademic tasks. Each night, write down everything you need to do on a piece of paper. Be specific as you write your list. Then prioritize your list and transfer this information into the time slots of your daily calendar (Table 12–1).

(✔) When Completed

9:00 – 9:30	
9:30 – 10:00	
10:00 – 10:30	
10:30 – 11:00	
11:00 – 11:30	
11:30 – 12:00	
12:00 – 12:30	
12:30 – 1:00	
1:00 – 1:30	
1:30 – 2:00	
2:00 – 2:30	
2:30 – 3:00	
3:00 – 3:30	
3:30 – 4:00	
4:00 – 4:30	
4:30 – 5:00	
5:00 – 5:30	
5:30 – 6:00	
6:00 – 6:30	
6:30 – 7:00	
7:00 – 7:30	
7:30 – 8:00	
8:00 – 8:30	
8:30 – 9:00	

FIGURE 12–3 A daily calendar.

TABLE 12–1   One student's To-Do List

To-Do List	Priortized To-Do List
Do grocery shopping	1. Attend English class
Go to post office	2. Read Chapter 7 in biology text
Read Chapter 7 in biology text	3. Do grocery shopping
Attend English class	4. Practice piano
Practice piano	5. Go to post office

Daily Calendar: Check when completed.

___11:00 – 12:00 English class
___2:00 – 2:30 Do grocery shopping
___2:30 – 3:00 Go to post office
___3:30 – 4:30 Practice piano
___5:00 – 6:30 Read Chapter 7 in biology text

EXERCISE 12–5

Directions: Write a to-do list. Prioritize your list and fill these items into the time slot on your daily calendar. Make a check mark next to each task that you complete.

ELIMINATING DISTRACTIONS

Students are often distracted. These distractions, <u>external</u> and <u>internal</u>, waste your time.

External Distractions

External distractions are elements in your surroundings that prevent you from accomplishing your goals. Some external distractions are the telephone, television, computer games, and excessive socializing. Staying on schedule will eliminate the <u>tendency</u> to allow these distractions from taking up too much of your time.

Internal Distractions

Internal distractions are your thoughts and feelings that interfere with your ability to concentrate.

The daily calendar will help you to eliminate internal distractions. You will focus on completing each task rather than wasting your time worrying about things that are out of your control. Sticking to a schedule keeps you organized and focused. Your concentration will improve.

MONITORING YOUR ABILITY TO MANAGE TIME

Managing time will help you to be a successful student. Once you have learned the strategies for managing time, you should stop and ask yourself whether these strategies are working for you. Ask yourself:

- Does my weekly schedule allow enough time for study?
- Am I still wasting too much time?
- Does my daily schedule allow me to take care of my important priorities?
- Am I meeting my semester goals?

AVOIDING PROCRASTINATION

If you are managing time, you will avoid <u>procrastination</u>, delaying what needs to be done. Do your work now—not later. Procrastination is the greatest source of anxiety for students. You will be more relaxed and your grades will improve if you don't procrastinae. Schedule your difficult assignments first, when your concentration is best. If you can discipline yourself to follow your schedule, you won't get into the habit of procrastination.

Managing your time will help you to be successful in <u>juggling</u> all your responsibilities at home, at work, and in school.

REVIEWING MANAGING TIME

TO LEARN	**USE THIS STRATEGY**
To set goals	Make a list of your semester goals.
To prioritize goals	Place your goals in order of importance to you.
To schedule	Use monthly, weekly, and daily calendars.
To eliminate distractions	Stay on schedule and concentrate on completing your tasks in order of importance.
To monitor your ability to manage time	Ask yourself whether your schedule is helping you to achieve your goals.
To avoid procrastination	Do work now—not later—stick to your schedule.

Chapter 13

Learning Active Listening Skills

LEARNING OBJECTIVES
VOCABULARY WORDS
VOCABULARY CHECK
UNDERSTANDING THE DIFFERENCE BETWEEN LISTENING AND HEARING
EVALUATING YOUR LISTENING HABITS
LEARNING STRATEGIES FOR ACTIVE LISTENING
MONITORING YOUR LISTENING COMPREHENSION
APPLYING ACTIVE LISTENING STRATEGIES TO SUCCESS IN SCHOOL
REVIEWING ACTIVE LISTENING SKILLS

LEARNING OBJECTIVES

In this chapter you will learn how to
- Evaluate your listening habits
- Monitor your listening comprehension
- Learn strategies for active listening
- Apply active listening strategies for success in school

VOCABULARY WORDS

The following vocabulary words are important to your understanding of the ideas in this chapter. These vocabulary words are <u>underscored</u> the first time they are used in the chapter. Read the list of words and definitions. Then check your understanding of these words before you read the chapter.

content the material to be learned in a course.
coworkers fellow employees.
distracted to have attention taken away.
interfere to get in the way of.

highlight emphasize.
journal an account of daily events.
objective lack of feeling toward or against.
passive not active.
rote use of memory without thought.
subject topic or area to be learned.

VOCABULARY CHECK

Directions: Choose the vocabulary word that best fits the sentence.

1. Catherine used a yellow marker to _____ the main ideas in her textbook.

2. My _____ and I have worked together for 5 years.

3. Math is my favorite _____.

4. Steven is easily _____ from his studies.

5. The English instructor assigned the class to write a _____ to keep a record of their daily activities.

6. Jonas didn't really understand the material, he learned it by _____.

7. 1 find the _____ of my chemistry course more difficult than I expected.

8. I wish you wouldn't _____ in my business.

9. Thelma is not _____ on this subject because she has strong feelings about this topic.

10. Wendy is _____ in class; she doesn't initiate any activity.

UNDERSTANDING THE DIFFERENCE BETWEEN LISTENING AND HEARING

Do you find that you have difficulty concentrating during class lectures? When you are working do you need to have your underline{coworkers} repeat instructions to you? Are you easily underline{distracted} when someone is speaking to you? If you have answered "yes" to these questions, you are hearing but not listening. When you are hearing, you are aware of sounds, but you are not interpreting these sounds into meaning. Listening involves comprehension. Listening is an active process. Hearing is underline{passive}. An active listener concentrates on and understands a speaker's main points. Your success in school and on the job is affected by your ability to be an active listener. You can learn how to focus your attention on a speaker's message.

EVALUATING YOUR LISTENING HABITS

One method of improving your listening skills is to evaluate your habits. Once you are aware of your listening problems, you can try to correct them. Eliminating bad listening habits will help you to learn important information in school and on the job.

Do you have any of the following listening problems?

_____ **Daydreaming.** Does your mind wander during class lectures? Do you find that you miss essential information before you come back to attention? Daydreaming is the most common listening problem. You can learn strategies to focus on a speaker's main ideas and keep your mind on the topic.

_____ **Pretending Attention.** Do you pretend to pay attention in class? Sometimes students are pretending to pay attention, but they are mentally asleep behind open eyes. When you are pretending attention, you are missing all the information. You are occupying a seat in class, but your mind is elsewhere.

_____ <u>Rote</u> **Note Taking.** Do you try to write every word instead of listening for your instructor's main points? When you are finished, you will end up with unfinished sentences and scrambled information. Rote note taking is a listening problem, because you are not focusing on the main ideas and important details.

_____ **Closing off the <u>Subject</u> or Speaker.** Do you turn off subjects or speakers without giving them a chance? Sometimes, you dislike a certain subject, and when you are required to take a course in this <u>content</u> area, you stop listening before the first class begins. Another problem occurs when you decide that you dislike your instructor before the semester begins. You might have heard negative things about this teacher from other students. However, you should be <u>objective</u>. Keep an open mind and give the instructor and the subject a chance. You will be surprised at how much you can learn if you give them your full attention.

_____ **Giving in to Distractions.** Do you get distracted easily? Do you let external noises, conversations, or events disturb you during class lessons? Sometimes, it is difficult to pay attention, but it is your responsibility as a listener to block out these distractions and to concentrate on your instructor's main ideas. Don't allow external distractions to <u>interfere</u> with your learning.

EXERCISE 13–1

Directions: Reread the list of five listening problems. Place a check next to any listening problem that you would like to improve.

LEARNING STRATEGIES FOR ACTIVE LISTENING

Now that you have recognized your listening problems, you can try to solve these problems by learning strategies for active listening.

To improve your listening concentration and comprehension,

- Listen for the main idea.
  Ask yourself: What is the topic of the lecture? What is the most important point being made about this topic?
- Listen for important details.
  Ask yourself: Which facts support the main idea?
- Paraphrase the information.
  Restate the speaker's ideas in your own words. Summarize the speakers message by asking the 5W questions.
  Who or **What** is the lecture about?_____
  What is the main point of the lecture? _____
  When? _____
  Where?_____
  Why or **How**?_____

MONITORING YOUR LISTENING COMPREHENSION

To monitor, or check, your active listening strategies, keep a listening <u>journal</u> for one week. This journal will help you keep track of your listening problems as they take place. You can then check to see if you did anything to correct your listening problem while you were in the situation. Did you remember to apply your active listening strategies? Did these strategies help to improve your concentration? Where you able to better understand your instructor's lecture? This listening journal will help you to check whether you are applying your active listening strategies.

As you can see from one student's listening journal (Fig. 13–1), the student is aware of listening problems and is now monitoring whether these problems were corrected.

EXERCISE 13–2

Directions: Fill in a listening journal (Fig. 13–2) for 1 week of classes. Monitor your listening comprehension. Then, evaluate your listening habits.

	Class	Type of listening problem	Did I apply listening strategies?	Was I able to paraphrase and summarize the information?
Monday	Biology	Pretending attention	No	No
Tuesday	English	Giving into distractions	Yes	Yes. Main point of lesson was how to revise an essay.
Wednesday	Computer	Closing off to speaker	No	No. I could not follow directions
Thursday	Math applications	Daydreaming	Yes	No. I already missed important information.
Friday	Part-time job	Closing off to subject	Yes	I understood the directions I had to follow to finish the job.

FIGURE 13–1 One student's listening journal.

Class	Type of listening problem	Did I apply listening strategies?	Was I able to paraphrase and summarize the information?
Monday			
Tuesday			
Wednesday			
Thursday			
Friday			

FIGURE 13–2 A listening journal.

APPLYING ACTIVE LISTENING STRATEGIES TO SUCCESS IN SCHOOL

Once you have learned active listening strategies, you can apply these strategies to improve your grades. You can be actively involved in improving your listening skills.

Are you physically and mentally prepared to pay attention in class? If you are tired or hungry, it is difficult to concentrate. Did you do your assignment? Class preparation makes you eager to listen. If you are unprepared, you probably feel uncomfortable and this discomfort interferes with concentration.

Pay attention to your instructor. Look directly at the speaker. Participate in class. Ask questions and listen for the answers. Sit in the front of the room if you have trouble seeing, hearing, or concentrating. Get involved in class discussions. Think about and react to the ideas discussed in class.

Applying active listening strategies will help you to take good notes in class. To take effective notes remember to:

- Listen for main ideas and important details.
- Paraphrase and summarize the information discussed in class.
- Pay extra attention to the instructor's introductory statements and summaries that <u>highlight</u> the most important ideas of the lesson.

Learning active listening strategies will help you to improve your grades. You will learn how to concentrate during class lessons, take better notes, and be actively involved in your success in school.

REVIEWING ACTIVE LISTENING SKILLS

TO LEARN	USE THIS STRATEGY
The difference between listening and hearing	Concentrate on and interpret the speaker's message.
How to evaluate your listening habits	Be aware of five listening problems:
	• Daydreaming
	• Pretending attention
	• Rote note taking
	• Closing off the subject or speaker
	• Giving in to distractions
Strategies for active listening	Listen for main ideas and important details. Paraphrase and summarize information.
To monitor your listening comprehension	Keep a listening journal.
To apply active listening strategies to success in school	Be prepared for listening physically and mentally. Take good notes.

Taking Notes

LEARNING OBJECTIVES

In this chapter you will learn how to
- Organize your notebook and notepaper
- Take notes from your textbook
- Take notes from your lectures
- Determine how many notes to take
- Take faster notes
- Study from your notes

VOCABULARY WORDS

The following vocabulary words are important to your understanding of the ideas in this chapter. These vocabulary words are <u>underscored</u> the first time they are used in the chapter. Read the list of words and definitions. Then check your understanding of these words before you read the chapter.

cardiac pertaining to the heart (Mosby's Dictionary, p. 300).

chronological arranged in order of time.

complement to complete or make perfect.

condensing making something more compact.

conventional traditional.

indentation the division of a document to create sections.

microcapillary tiny vessel connecting arterioles and venules.

molecules the smallest units that exhibit the properties of an element or compound (Mosby's Dictonary, p. 1216).

portable able to be carried easily.

venipuncture the transcutaneous puncture of a vein by a sharp rigid stylet or cannula carrying a flexible plastic catheter or by a steel needle attached to a syringe or catheter (Mosby's Dictionary, 7th ed, p. 1948).

VOCABULARY CHECK

Directions: Choose the vocabulary word that best fits into the sentence.

1. A clearly written textbook will _____ a good lecture.

2. To draw blood you need to _____ a vein.

3. The elderly patient died from a _____ arrest.

4. A part of the circulatory system is a _____.

5. When she took brief notes from the lengthy textbook, she was _____ many of the author's ideas.

6. The smaller medical text was more _____ than the larger one.

7. He wrote his entire life history in _____ order.

8. In their chemistry class, the students studied _____ under a very powerful microscope.

9. The _____ of less important ideas was achieved with many margins.

10. The old-fashioned teacher held many _____ ideas about teaching.

IMPORTANCE OF TAKING GOOD NOTES

Your success as a health care student depends almost entirely on how well you take notes from your textbooks and lectures. When it comes to preparing for tests, you must have textbook and lecture notes that adequately record the information you need to learn. Few people have the time to reread the vast amount of material from the textbook to prepare for a midterm or final examination. Few people have the ability to catch and remember every word spoken in a lecture. That is why it is important to have strategies for taking good notes from your books and lectures. You must learn to focus only on the information that is important. You do not want to waste your time recording and remembering facts that may not be necessary to learn. Knowing the strategies for taking good notes will not only save you time but will also enhance your test taking skills.

EXERCISE 14–1

Directions: Below is a checklist for determining how good your present note-taking system is. Check "Yes" or "No."

1. Do I have background knowledge of the textbook or lecture subject?

   Yes _____ No _____

2. Do I see any connection between textbook notes and lecture notes?

   Yes _____ No _____

3. Do I keep current with all my reading assignments?

   Yes _____ No _____

4. Do I attend all lectures?

   Yes _____ No _____

5. Is my notebook well organized?

   Yes _____ No _____

6. Do I have a system for setting up the notebook sheets of paper?

   Yes _____ No _____

7. Do I know how much information to write or highlight?

   Yes _____ No _____

8. Can I tell important facts from unimportant facts?

   Yes _____ No _____

9. Do I take speedy notes?

   Yes _____ No _____

10. Do I have strategies for studying notes?

    Yes _____ No _____

If you answered "no" to most of these questions, you need to learn strategies for taking better notes. This chapter will teach you the strategies for organizing, taking, and studying textbook and lecture notes.

USING YOUR NOTES SUCCESSFULLY

Some students feel it is okay to take notes from their textbooks and lectures and then ignore them until test time. Other students, however, realize that to get good grades you must constantly review your notes. These students realize that textbook notes and lecture notes are interconnected. In order to get the best grades, they use the following strategies:

- Before lectures, take and review textbook notes on the subject of the lecture. This will build your background knowledge of the topic, and the lecture will be that much more understandable.
- After the lecture, review your textbook notes again. This will reinforce your learning the information.
- Before test time, study both the lecture notes and the textbook notes until they are fully learned. This is good test preparation.

TIME MANAGEMENT AND NOTE TAKING

An important aspect to good note taking is time management. This means allowing sufficient time for reading your textbooks and attending all lectures.

- Stay current. Do not fall behind in your textbook reading. You may be responsible for textbook information on exams and once you are behind, you may never be able to catch up. Maintain your scheduling calendars and keep pace with your reading assignments.
- Attend all lectures. Having to borrow someone else's notes is never as good as taking them yourself. If possible, ignore minor physical and emotional upsets and get into the habit of attending all your classes.
- Arrive early for your lectures. This will give you time to organize your notebook for good note taking. Also, you do not want to miss the beginning of the lecture. Many instructors introduce their main points at the very beginning of the class period, so this is something you may not want to skip.

CHOOSING YOUR NOTEBOOK

The first practical step for taking good textbook and lecture notes is buying and setting up your notebook. This will depend on personal preference. The main thing to keep in mind, however, is to organize your notebook so that each subject is kept separated from the other subjects. This may mean buying different 8 × 11 inch spiral notebooks for each subject or spiral notebooks that are divided into three to five sections. The advantage to using spiral notebooks is that they are lightweight and easy to carry. Also, you need to bring only the spiral notebook that is used for a particular daily class. The disadvantage to using a spiral notebook is that you may run out of paper. The manufacturer of these notebooks cannot anticipate how many pages you will actually need. You may find yourself having to buy more than one spiral notebook for each subject. This may prove bothersome and confusing.

An alternative to a spiral notebook is a hard cover loose-leaf binder. If this is your choice, be sure to buy the colorful dividers to keep each of your subjects separate. The advantage to using a loose-leaf binder is that you can control the number of pages for each subject section. If you use more paper in one class than in another, you can always insert more lined paper in that section. The disadvantage to using loose-leaf binders is that, depending on the type, they are not so <u>portable</u>. They may be heavy to carry and may not fit so well into your book bag or backpack. However, you can now purchase for each of your subjects an inexpensive lightweight loose-leaf notebook. Be aware, though, that there is always the possibility that the rings will not close right or will open at the wrong time, and that can mean disarranged or lost notes.

Whatever your preference in notebooks, remember that you must keep notes from each of your subjects separate and distinct from the other subjects. You may also want to consider using different notebooks for lecture notes and textbook notes. Again, the choice is yours.

EXERCISE 14–2

Directions: Think back over your past school years and try to remember whether you used spiral notebooks or loose-leaf binders. In the space below, write some of the advantages or disadvantages you may have found using one type of notebook or another. Use the list as a guide to help you decide which style of notebook is right for you.

_____

_____

_____

_____

ORGANIZING YOUR NOTEPAPER

Whether you are taking textbook or lecture notes, it is important to set up your notepaper in a way that will make your notes understandable when you read them days or weeks later. To organize your lecture notepaper, you must arrive in class a few minutes early to prepare your paper. To organize your textbook notes, plan to begin each study session with setting up your notepapers.

The first strategy to use in organizing your notepaper is numbering and putting the current date on top of each paper. This is important when it comes time to study for exams. By numbering and dating each page, you will know which notes are needed for a specific exam period. You will know which notes to study. Also, if your notes should accidentally get loose, you will have a way of reorganizing them. Keeping your notes in numerical and <u>chronological</u> order is the best way of ensuring that your notes are well organized.

Spiral Notebook

Loose-leaf Binder

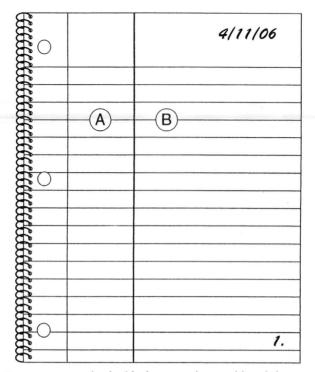

Figure 14–1 Notepaper organized with date, number, and hand-drawn second margin.

The next strategy for organizing your notepaper is to draw a line down the page, about an inch and a half from the red left-hand margin (see Fig. 14–1). When taking textbook or lecture notes, leave this space empty. (Note area A in Fig. 14–1.) All your notes should be written in the area marked "B" in Figure 14–1. Later you will write in the area marked "A" if you need to add any information you missed, create headings, or jot down comments and observations you believe are necessary to finish your notes. Organizing your notepaper in this manner will ensure that your notes are complete and useful for test preparation.

EXERCISE 14–3

Directions: At your next lecture or study period, practice organizing your notepaper with the number, date, and second left-hand margin. Then respond to the following statements by checking "Yes" or "No."

1. My notes appear to be better organized now that I number and date them.

   Yes _____No_____

2. My notes look neater now that I use the second margin for additional notes.

   Yes _____No_____

3. It is easier to add new information to my notes now that I have the second margin.

   Yes _____No_____

4. It is more convenient studying for exams now that I organize my notes with numbers, date, and the second left-hand margin.

   Yes _____No_____

If you answer "Yes" to most of these questions, these strategies for organizing your notepaper are right for you. Continue to use these methods for all your health care classes.

If you answer "No" to most of these questions, keep using these strategies until your next exam. You may be pleasantly surprised to see better test results.

TAKING NOTES FROM YOUR TEXTBOOK

As you probably realize by now, your time as a health care student is very precious. This means that you must use your limited amount of time sensibly. When it comes to reading assignments, you may feel overwhelmed because there is so much to read with so little time to do it in. When it comes to preparing for exams, you do not have the time to reread all the assigned chapters. Therefore you need strategies for taking good notes from your textbook for test preparation. Good textbook notes not only will save you time when you are getting ready for tests but will probably result in better test scores. The two strategies for taking textbook notes are

- Highlighting
- Margin writing

HIGHLIGHTING

Highlighting information in your textbook is probably the most popular way of condensing information in your textbook. To highlight important facts, you use a pen, pencil, or special highlighting marker and underline all the sentences you think are meaningful for learning the subject matter. The advantage to using the highlighting strategy is that it saves time. You do not have to rewrite information that is already written. Highlighting is quick and, when done properly, is probably the most efficient way of taking notes from a textbook. The disadvantage to highlighting is that most students tend to overdo it. You have no doubt seen a page in a textbook that is totally highlighted with a yellow marker. What is the point to highlighting every word on the page? The effectiveness of the highlighting strategy is that it is supposed to direct your eyes to only the most important words and ideas on the page. Therefore you must highlight only the most significant facts. To do this, you can use the heading strategy discussed in Chapter 5, Reading The Textbook. To review this strategy,

- Look at the boldfaced headings on each page.
- Turn each boldfaced heading into a question.
- Highlight only those facts that answer the heading question.

Following is an example from *The Medical Assistant: Administrative and Clinical* by Kinn, Woods, and Derge (p. 194) of how a health care student used the heading strategy to guide her highlighting. Notice that she underlined only the facts that answered her heading question.

Example 14–1

CONSULTATION REPORTS

- What are consultation reports?

<u>Physicians who act as consultants</u> are expected to <u>prepare a detailed report of their findings and recommendations and send it to the referring physicians.</u> The *consultation report* is <u>dictated by the consulting physician</u> to be transcribed within the office or by an independent transcriptionist if outside services are used. The consultation <u>report</u> is frequently <u>quite long</u>, and <u>promptness in preparations is important</u>.

EXERCISE 14–4

Directions: Below is an excerpt from Flynn's *Procedures in Phlebotomy* (p. 80-81). Turn the heading into a question and highlight the facts that answer your question. Remember to stay focused on the question and do not highlight too much. You can use a pen, pencil, or highlighting marker.

BLOOD LANCETS

For difficult patients and in situations that normally call for microcapillary techniques, a blood lancet may be used. This is a small, sterile, disposable instrument used for skin puncture. Semiautomated lancets are available with a variety of point lengths to help control the depth of puncture, which is especially important in children and infants. A variety of semiautomated lancet devices are commercially available, and although the manual lancet was the most commonly used device for microcapillary puncture in the past, the semi-automated devices are now more commonly employed.

MARGIN WRITING

To complement your highlighting of the important points in your textbook, you may also want to consider writing in the margins of your textbook. Following is a list of suggested items that you may use for margin writing:

- *Headings:* You can divide lengthy passages into more manageable sections by creating your own headings. Write these headings between paragraphs or in the margin where you want to divide the passage.
- *Summaries:* You can summarize or condense lengthy passages into brief summaries by writing in the margins of your book. You will not be able to be wordy because of the limited space. Your margin summaries should cover only the most important information in the passage.
- *Symbols:* Using various symbols can be an easy way of emphasizing important facts from the textbook. Some useful symbols are "T" to show what details your instructor said will appear on tests; "B" to show what information in your textbook corresponds to information your instructor wrote on the board during a lecture; and "R" to designate those sections in the textbook that your teacher may have read aloud and discussed in class. Using symbols like these will help you connect important ideas from your lecture to the material in your textbook.

Following is an example from a textbook by Flynn (pp. 38-39). Notice how one student used headings, summaries, and symbols to emphasize important points in the textbook.

Example 14–2

The Digestive System

Food must be broken down into small <u>molecules</u> so that it can be digested, absorbed, and metabolized by the body. The digestive system is responsible for these functions. After food is ingested, chewed, and swallowed, it moves down the esophagus into the stomach. Gastric glands in the stomach secrete gastric juice, which is composed of hydrochloric acid, mucus, enzymes, and other fluids. Food particles mix with these and are then emptied into the small intestine by peristalsis.

B.
Peristalsis is the rhythmic wave of smooth muscle contraction. It is here, in the small intestine, that digestion is completed. Intestinal enzymes and products produced by the liver, gallbladder, and pancreas are required elements to aid in this process. The liver produces bile, which is concentrated and stored in the gallbladder until needed. Bile contains bile salts, which help in the digestion of fat molecules. The pancreas produces enzymes such as amylase and lipase, which help to break down complex carbohydrates and fatty acids. Nutrients are then absorbed, and the remainder is passed on to the large intestine.

R.
Absorption occurs by active transport across cell membranes through villi that line the inner surface of the small intestine. Each villus contains a blood capillary and a lymphatic capillary (lacteal). Simple sugars and amino acids pass into the blood capillaries, and fatty acids enter the lacteals. In the large intestine, water and electrolytes are absorbed, and waste products are excreted via the rectum and anus.

After nutrients are absorbed, they are utilized by the body to produce energy for all the chemical *T.* reactions that occur. These chemical reactions are called metabolism. Metabolic reactions are divided into *T.* two categories: anabolism and catabolism. Anabolism is the process of making larger molecules from *T.* smaller ones. This requires the use of chemical energy or ATP. Catabolism is the breakdown of large *B.* molecules into smaller ones. Energy is released during catabolism. Gastroenterology is the study of the *B.* digestive organs. A gastrologist studies diseases of the stomach.

Digestion (margin note)

Absorption (margin note)

Metabolism (margin note)

EXERCISE 14–5

Directions: In the following passage from Young and Kennedy (p. 167-168), practice emphasizing important details by creating headings, summaries, and symbols. Refer to Example 14–2 if you need help.

COMPUTER SCHEDULING

The computer has replaced the appointment book in many practices. Software for appointment scheduling ranges from relatively simple programs that merely display available and scheduled times to more sophisticated systems. Many programs can display such information as the length and type of appointment required and day or time preferences. The computer can then select the best appointment time based on the information entered into the computer.

The computer can also be used to keep track of future appointments. For example, when a patient calls and inquires about an appointment, the system can search by his or her name to find the time and date. Printouts can also run to show the physician's daily schedule, including the patients' names and telephone numbers and the reason for the visit. Multiple copies of these schedules can be made, according to the needs of the practice.

One advantage of computer scheduling is that more than one person can access the system at one time, and the information is available to all operators. The medical assistant can generate a hard copy of the next day's appointments before leaving each evening. In some facilities, employees still maintain an appoitment book as a backup to computer scheduling.

TAKING NOTES FROM YOUR LECTURES

As was mentioned earlier, it is impossible to take down all of the instructor's words during a lecture. You must concentrate on the main ideas and the important details (see Chapters 1 and 2). You should also write down the important information in such a way that days later you will be able to tell at a glance what is the main idea and what is a detail. You can do this by using the <u>indentation</u> strategy. The main ideas should be written next to the second margin and the important details should be indented or written in a few letters to the right. See Figure 14–2.

EXERCISE 14–6

Directions: Following is a selection from LaFleur-Brooks and Gillingham, *Health Unit Coordinating,* p. 434. Using the selection as a lecture, take notes on the sheet of notebook paper on the following page. If it is a main idea, start writing close to the second margin. If it is an important detail, indent. You may want to consider taking notes on less important details and indenting them even more.

Two **medical emergencies**—that is, life-threatening situations—that require remaining calm, swift action, and good communication by the health unit coordinator are **cardiac arrest** and **respiratory arrest**. (It is common hospital terminology to refer to these as *code arrests.) The hospital telephone operator is notified immediately to announce the code. In a cardiac arrest the patient's heart contractions are absent or grossly insufficient, and there is no pulse and no blood pressure. In respiratory arrest, the patient may* cease to breathe or the respirations become so depressed that the patient does not receive oxygen to sustain life. Both conditions require quick action by hospital personnel and the use of emergency equipment. Treatment must be instituted within 3 to 4 minutes, because the brain cells deteriorate rapidly from lack of oxygen.

Each hospital nursing unit and department maintains a code or crash cart. This is taken to the code arrest patient's room immediately. It is important for the health unit coordinator to know the location of the code or crash cart and any other emergency equipment so that it can be brought quickly to their nursing unit when needed.

Hospitals have designated hospital personnel who report each code arrest. They are members of the code arrest team. They may be employed in various hospital departments,

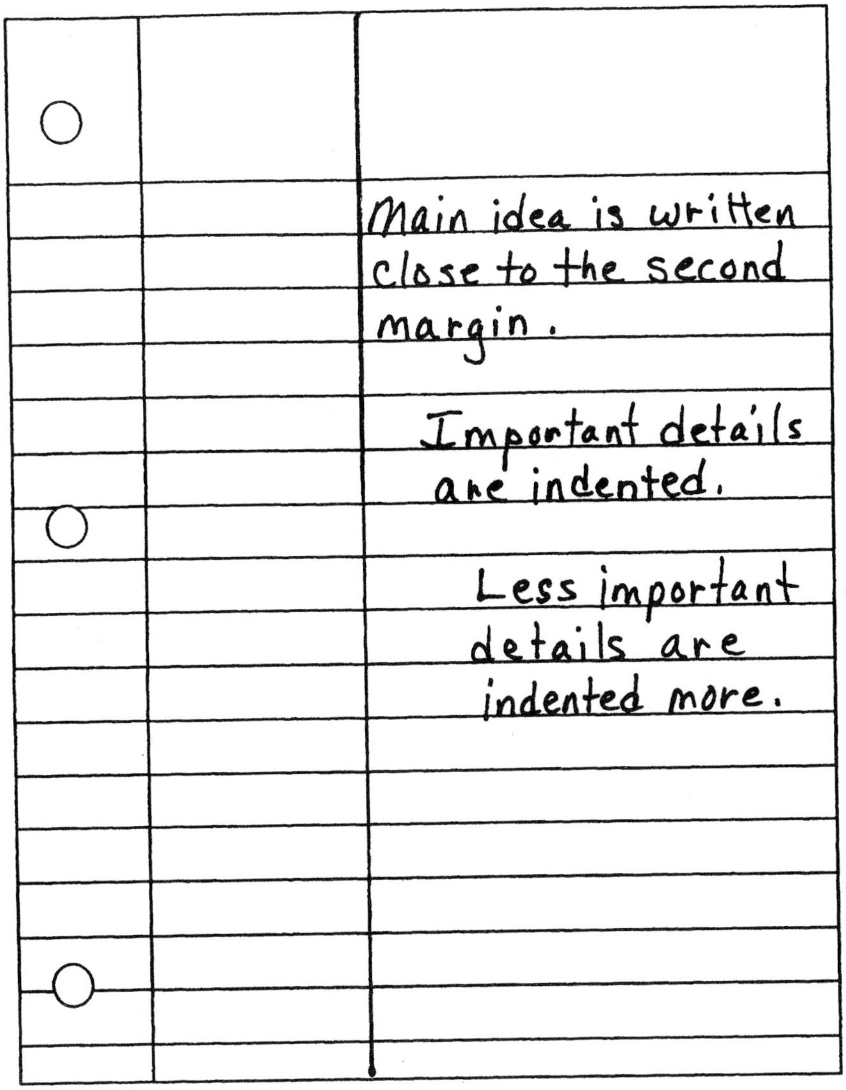

Main idea is written close to the second margin.

Important details are indented.

Less important details are indented more.

FIGURE 14–2   Indentation strategy

such as intensive or coronary care, other nursing units, the respiratory care department, pulmonary function department, surgery, and so forth.

Instructors' Cues

Now that you have a system for taking lecture notes, you are left with the decision of determining what information is important to record. Fortunately, your instructor will willingly or unwillingly provide you with cues that should let you know what ideas are significant. By recognizing these cues, you will know what facts to write in your notes and possibly what facts to leave out. Following are the cues most instructors give to indicate meaningful material.

- **Ideas Written on the Board:** Make sure you copy any information the teacher writes on the board. As mentioned earlier, you may want to indicate these facts with a "B" for board in your notes.

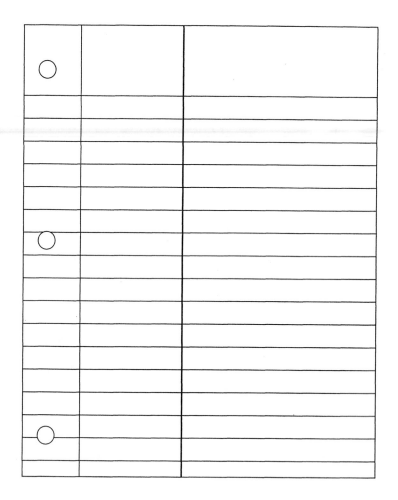

- **Verbal Tips:** You may be fortunate to have an instructor who will say, "this will be on the test" or "these are important ideas." Make sure you write these facts accurately and mark these notes with a "T" for test or an "I" for important.
- **Numbering Ideas:** Many teachers may introduce important points by numbering them. They do this by saying "first," "second," "third," etc. If your teacher goes to the trouble of numbering ideas, you should consider them important enough to copy in your notebook.
- **Body Language:** Some instructors will make their voices louder or gesture with their hands to indicate important ideas. Stay alert to these or other body signs that the teacher will use to suggest important ideas.

At the end of the lecture, resist the temptation to stop listening and gather your books. Many times the instructor will summarize the important points at the end of the lecture, so pay attention and stay put until the teacher finishes talking.

HOW MANY NOTES TO TAKE

Many students are puzzled about how many notes they should be writing from their textbooks and lectures. The best strategy in this matter is to know the course requirements and let that help you determine how much to write. If the course deals with broad concepts, you probably will be held responsible for fewer or less detailed notes. If the course presents more factual information, you will need to write greater and more detailed notes.

The best way to determine the requirements of the course is to read the description in the course catalogue, talk with other students who have taken the course, or speak with the instructor directly. Getting this information while the semester is just beginning will help you determine how many notes you should be taking.

FASTER NOTE TAKING

Many people feel that they would be more successful students if they were able to take lecture notes more quickly. They express frustration at not being able to "catch" all the important points being taught in the classroom. They claim they would do better on tests if their notes were complete. By learning the strategies for faster note taking—streamlining your handwriting and abbreviating and using symbols—these students will improve the rate of their note taking and become better students.

Streamlining Your Handwriting

To take notes more quickly, it is sometimes necessary to make changes in your handwriting. Your note-taking rate will improve if you write in script rather than in printing. When you write in script, one letter connects to the other so that the flow of your writing is faster. However, when you use script, make sure you eliminate any unnecessary strokes or curlicues. Your ability to use a plain streamlined script will greatly enhance your lecture note-taking skills. Following are examples of too fancy a script and a streamlined script.

Streamline your handwriting

Streamline your handwriting

EXERCISE 14–7

Directions: Below is a short excerpt from Solomon, *Introduction to Human Anatomy and Physiology*, p. 47. Using it to substitute for a lecture, rewrite it in your usual handwriting in the space provided. Time yourself. If you see that your handwriting is too elaborate, try rewriting it in a more streamlined fashion. Time yourself again. Notice whether your timing has improved.

The skeleton found in science laboratories consists of dry, dead bones. In contrast, the bone, cartilage, and other connective tissues of the skeletal system in a living body are active, living tissues. Their cells must have nutrients, oxygen, and energy; they carry on metabolism, they produce waste products, some aspects of their metabolism is regulated by hormones, and they function closely with the muscular system.

Time for first try:_____

Time for second try:_____

Abbreviating and Using Symbols

Another strategy for faster note taking is to use abbreviations or symbols to replace common words. It is much quicker to write "&" for "and" or to spell "patient" "pat." You can use conventional abbreviations and symbols, or you can make up your own. If you make up your own, be sure you remember their meanings. It will do you little good if you use a symbol or abbreviation that you can't understand a few weeks later when you prepare for an exam. Following is a selection adapted from Flynn, p. 129. Note how one student used abbreviations and symbols to create a type of shorthand system for taking notes quickly.

Example 14–3

The glucose tolerance test (GTT) is done on individuals who are being screened for hyperglycemia, also
known as **diabetes mellitus**. The test is also used to screen for **hypoglycemia**. The purpose of the test
is to determine the patient's blood glucose level after the patient consumes a fixed amount of glucose
(usually 100 gm). The test takes from 3 to 5 hours. Although there is nothing unique about the actual
collection process itself, the number of venipunctures performed in a relatively short period makes this
test significant.

After a patient has fasted for at least 12 hours, a blood sample is collected using routine collection
procedures. The blood may be collected in a plain tube (without any anticoagulant) or in a tube
especially designed to preserve glucose levels (such as a gray-stoppered tube with sodium fluoride and
potassium oxalate).

EXERCISE 14–8

Directions: The following is a passage from McCurnin, *Clinical Textbook for Veterinary Technicians*, p. 707. Write your own system of abbreviations and symbols in the space between the lines. At the beginning of your next lesson, check to see if you can decode your own system of abbreviations and symbols.

The two methods for gloving yourself are *closed gloving* and *open gloving*. The risk of contamination is minimized with closed gloving since the outside of the gloves never contacts skin. There is a much higher risk of contamination during open gloving, and it is generally reserved for minor procedures when a gown is not worn (e.g., sterile patient scrub, urinary catheterization).

TAPING YOUR LECTURES

Another strategy for ensuring well-written notes is to tape your lectures with a portable audiocassette recorder. However, before you attempt to do this, get your instructor's permission; some people feel uncomfortable when they know they are being taped. The advantages to taping your lectures are many. First, during your study period you can replay the tape and fill in any missing information. Second, listening to your lectures over and over again is a good strategy for test preparation. Third, you can listen to your lecture tape anytime—as you drive to classes, when you are commuting to school, or at your leisure at home. And, finally, you can have a friend tape a lecture for you if you cannot attend class.

Make sure that your recorder is easy to carry and battery operated. Always remember to carry extra batteries. Buy the long-running blank cassette tapes and sit up front, close to the instructor, so you can get a clear recording. You want your lecture tapes to be as distinct as possible.

STUDYING FROM YOUR NOTES

After a lecture, as soon as you can, review your notes for completeness. This may mean listening to your tape or consulting with a fellow student. Once you feel your notes are as thorough as possible, you should begin to learn these notes in a systematic manner. A wonderful strategy for learning notes is to use the heading method.

Creating Headings

Just as your textbook passages are divided by headings, so should your class notes be divided by headings. Decide where in your notes there is a topic change and, using a different color pen, put in a heading. To create the topic, ask yourself what is this passage mostly about. The answer will be the topic and will work well for a heading. Do this for all the pages in your notebook.

Once you have made headings for all the different topics in your notes, turn these headings into questions. When you are studying for an exam, focus on the information in your notes that will answer the heading question. Below is an example of how a student created headings and questions and highlighted only the important information that answered the heading question.

Example 14–4

- What is this passage mostly about?
- Influenza = Topic = Heading
- What is influenza = Heading question

Influenza virus A produces the most serious form of influenza, with <u>symptoms of fever, chills, headache, myalgia, sore throat, and cough.</u> The <u>onset of symptoms</u> is approximately <u>1 to 4 days after contact</u> with infected respiratory secretions. <u>Infected persons shed the virus for 24 hours before the onset of symptoms and for 3 to 4 days during the course of the disease.</u> Death associated with this virus is usually the result of primary influenza pneumonia or a secondary bacterial pneumonia. The influenza viruses that are the cause of epidemics and nosocomial outbreaks change from season to season, and a new vaccine is manufactured each year (Flynn, p. 66).

EXERCISE 14–9

Directions: Following is a passage from Diehl, *Medical Transcription: Techniques and Procedures*, p. 179. After carefully reading the passage, determine the topic and use it for the heading. Turn the heading into a question and highlight only those facts from the passage that answer the heading question.

When copy is prepared for printing, it is corrected and marked, with correction symbols placed either in the margin or between the lines to indicate the changes to be made.

In proofreading your own copy, you may be more informal, using marginal notes when there is no room on the single-spaced copy to indicate the change.

While you are a student, your instructor will proofread your work and may mark the copy and use marginal notes in a variety of ways. Therefore, let us examine the proofreading marks as they are used formally and see how we may modify them for our own use. Your instructor may wish to add his or her marking symbols as well.

Other Strategies for Studying Your Notes

You may believe that preparing for an exam means reading and rereading your notes. However, you may have had the experience of sitting at your desk, hour after hour, and "spacing out" when you should have been focusing on your textbook or lecture notes. You probably discovered at test time that all you accomplished was wasting time. Successful students are those who have discovered that more active strategies are necessary for quality test preparation. This means more active note-learning strategies.

An excellent strategy for using your notes to prepare for a test is to create quizzes. At the end of an evening's studying, and before you close the books, make up a quiz covering that day's materials. At the beginning of your next homework session, take the quiz and see how well you have done. Another good studying strategy is to make up a chart of all the information you need to learn. Make a second chart, omitting most of the information except for some guiding facts and try to fill in the chart without looking at the original. Also use your tape recorder and play back the lecture when you are washing dishes or sorting socks. Finally, make flash cards of the important vocabulary words. Print the word on one side of an index card and its definition on the other side. During your study time, look at the word and try to recall the definition. Or, for more variety, look at the definition and try to remember the word. Being creative about taking and studying textbook and lecture notes will go a long way to making you a more successful student.

REVIEWING THE LEARNING STRATEGIES

TO LEARN	USE THIS STRATEGY
Successful use of notes	Time management
	Careful choice of notebook
	Notepaper organizing
Note taking from textbook	Highlighting
	Margin writing
Note taking from lectures	Indenting
	Interpreting instructor's cues
Length of notes	Learning requirements of course
Faster note taking	Streamlining handwriting
	Abbreviating and using symbols
	Taping lectures
Note studying	Creating headings
	Creating questions
	Making quizzes
	Making charts
	Listening to lecture tapes
	Making flash cards

Chapter
15

Improving Test Scores

LEARNING OBJECTIVES

In this chapter you will learn how to
- Improve your test scores
- Use five strategies to help you prepare for and take tests more successfully

VOCABULARY WORDS

The following vocabulary words are important to your understanding of the ideas in this chapter. These vocabulary words are <u>underscored</u> the first time they are used in the chapter. Read the list of words and definitions. Then check your understanding of these words before you read the chapter.

ethicists persons who study morality.

gastrointestinal pertaining to the stomach and intestine.

host an animal or plant that harbors and provides sustenance for another organism.

hypotension lowered blood pressure.

mobilize to put into action.

obligation a commitment to acting in certain ways.

opponents those who disagree.

radiation energy carried by waves or a stream of particles.

transmission passage or transfer of a disease from one person to another.

utility usefulness.

VOCABULARY CHECK

Directions: Choose the vocabulary word that best fits into the sentence.

1. She was suffering from _____, so the doctor gave her medication to raise her blood pressure.

2. The student felt an _____ to study and pass the course.

3. The mechanic was concerned with the _____ of the new tool.

4. Sometimes it is difficult to _____ people to work at improving their environment.

5. A hazard of too much _____ is a severe burn.

6. The scientist was concerned about the _____ of the disease to a new population.

7. The _____ was concerned with the moral issues of the plan.

8. The disease went from a source to a _____.

9. The _____ of the new plan argued for their own point of view.

10. Her stomach pain was caused by a _____ infection.

HOW TO IMPROVE YOUR TEST SCORES

The purpose of tests is evaluation. Tests allow you, the student, and your instructor to find out what you have learned and what you still need to learn.

Of course, students worry about test grades. Doing well on tests is every student's goal. You can learn strategies to improve your grades. However, these strategies have to be applied long before the date of the exam.

Strategy 1: Plan Ahead

Your instructor will assign test dates in advance. Apply your time-management skills. Find out the assignments you need to study for the exam. Make sure that you know which information from your readings, lectures, or labs will be on the test. Then use your monthly, weekly, and daily calendars to schedule enough study time for your exam.

Many students in the health fields are juggling school with busy work and family schedules. Finding time to study can be a problem. Therefore organization is essential. Use your calendars to plan your study time. Stick to your schedule. Don't procrastinate! Avoiding your work today means doing a double assignment the next day.

Cramming, trying to prepare for an exam at the last minute, is not a successful strategy. Cramming increases anxiety. This nervousness often interferes with your test performance.

Do you understand how to plan ahead to schedule enough time to study for tests? Yes_____   No_____

Strategy 2: Keep Up with Assignments

Assignments should be done on a regular basis. Keep up with all the reading on your class syllabus. Don't fall behind.

Be an active reader. As you read your assignments, **remember** to be an **active reader.** **Preview** the reading material. **Ask** questions. **Write** summaries and outlines. **Learn** the new **vocabulary** that helps you to understand the ideas in each chapter. Pay attention to **illustrations** and **formulas**.

Do you remember to use your active reading strategies when reading home assignments? Yes _____   No _____

Use Active Listening and Effective Note-taking Strategies. Be prepared for each class session. Don't skip classes. Regular attendance is necessary if you are to understand a sequence of information. In the health fields, details are important. Take accurate notes. Apply active listening strategies. Pay attention to all main ideas and details highlighted in each lecture or lab. Ask questions if you don't understand the material presented. Summarize or outline the material presented in class.

Do you concentrate during class lectures? Yes _____   No _____
Do your class notes help you study for tests? Yes _____   No _____

Strategy 3: Study and Learn Material

Even if you have attended every class and read every assignment, you still have to study before every test.

- Review all class notes, summaries, outlines, and underlined material from your textbooks periodically throughout the course. **Don't cram!**
- Organize information into categories. It will be easier for you to remember organized material.
- Review vocabulary. Definitions are important in helping you learn information in the health fields. In fact, it is helpful to keep a notebook of the words and definitions that are highlighted in each chapter. Some students prefer keeping words and definitions on 3 × 5 inch index cards. Learn these definitions before the test.
- Pay attention to illustrations and formulas. Make sure that you understand how these pictures and numbers relate to the ideas in the chapter.
- Use mnemonics, a technique for improving the memory, to help you learn formulas, definitions, or ideas in the text. Mnemonic devices are easily

remembered words, sentences, or rhymes that help you to remember more difficult information. Mnemonic devices work by association and help you to remember information that is difficult to organize. Some common mnemonic devices are

Rhymes
    i before e except after c
    or when sounding like a
    as in neighbor and weigh
Acronyms - a word made from the initial letter of the parts of the information to be
        remembered.
    HOMES - to remember the five Great Lakes
    H - Huron
    O - Ontario
    M - Michigan
    E - Erie
    S - Superior

Try to create mnemonic devices to help you remember information.

Do you find mnemonics a helpful memory tool? Yes _____No _____

- Don't accept not understanding. Don't give up. Monitor your learning. When you don't understand information, try another approach to learning. Make sure that your study schedule allows you time to ask your instructor or other students to explain difficult ideas to you **before** the test.
- Find out how you learn best. Do you remember information by listening, reading, writing, or discussing the material? Do you find a combination of these methods most effective for learning? Use the learning style that works best for you.
- Design practice tests. Ask your instructor if the test questions will be objective, essay, or both. Answer the questions at the end of each chapter in your textbook.
- Check your answers. Then make up a practice test. Close your book and answer your own test questions. Correct your test. What do you know? What do you still have to learn? Students find that questions on their practice tests often turn up on the actual exam.

List those techniques that you think will help you to study and learn information:

_____

_____

_____

_____

Strategy 4: Take the Test Successfully

Learning how to take a test can improve your test scores. Whether your test is objective or essay, use these strategies:

- Read the test directions carefully before you answer any questions.
- Understand the grading system. Spend extra time on questions that are worth more points.

- Keep track of time.
- Answer the questions that you are sure of first. Then go back to questions that are more difficult for you.
- Answer the questions asked.
- Save time at the end to review your test and make any corrections or additions.
- Write clearly.

Taking Objective Tests

Objective tests are those with multiple-choice, short-answer, matching, or true-false questions. To do well on objective tests, you should learn how to answer four types of questions: multiple-choice, short-answer, matching, and true-false.

LEARNING HOW TO ANSWER MULTIPLE CHOICE QUESTIONS

When you answer multiple-choice questions, you select one answer from several choices. The following strategies will help you learn how to select the correct answer.

- Statements that contain words like *always*, *every*, *never*, and *all* are usually too broad. They are often incorrect.
- If two choices have the same meaning, they are both incorrect. Therefore, you eliminate both these choices when you select your answer.
- Be aware of directional words such as *but, except*, and *however*. They signal opposite meanings.
- To answer multiple-choice questions, you need to know how to:
  - Find the main ideas
  - Find and remember details that support the main idea
  - Draw conclusions
  - Learn vocabulary meanings through context

Example 15–1 ───────────────

Directions: Read the following excerpt adapted from a health care textbook (Diehl, p. 44). Answer the multiple-choice questions based on the selection. Then read the explanation of the answers.

WORD WRAP

A feature in which a word that has more characters than will fit at the end of a line is automatically moved to the beginning of the next line. It increases speed by eliminating the need for using the enter key at the end of each line.

1. Word wrap
   a. is automatic
   b. moves every word to the beginning of each line
   c. just drops the cursor
   d. automatically lifts up to the line above
2. Word wrap moves a word
   a. next to the right margin
   b. to the beginning of each page
   c. to the beginning of the next line
   d. past the left margin

3. Word wrap
   a. increases the number of lines on a computer screen
   b. decreases typing speed
   c. eliminates typing
   d. increases typing speed

The correct answer to number 1 is choice (a). The word *every* in choice (b) makes that answer incorrect. The word *just* in answer (c) eliminates that choice. The answer (d) says *up* and *above* while the text says *down*.

The correct answer to number 2 is choice (c). The answer is *to the next line* not *next to the right margin*. Therefore choice (a) is incorrect. Choice (b) is incorrect because the correct choice is *line* not *page*. The word *left* in choice (d) eliminates that answer choice.

The correct answer to number 3 is (d). Choice (a) is incorrect because the *typing speed* is *increased* not *the number of lines*. The word *decreases* in choice (b) eliminates that choice. The information in choice (c) is incorrect. Typing is not *eliminated*; typing speed is increased.

Answering multiple-choice questions requires careful attention to detail in reading the passage, the questions, and the choices.

EXERCISE 15–1

Directions: Read the following excerpt from a health care text (Young and Kennedy, p. 201). Answer the multiple-choice questions based on the selection. Use the strategies you learned for answering multiple-choice questions.

Computers. Computers have made composing correspondence simple. Various letters and documents may be saved and reused time after time by changing the name and basic information contained within the text. Computers can add graphics to text, compute figures, and use multimedia in communications—all of which enhance the appearance and effectiveness of the document.

Word Processors. Word Processors are used mainly for letter writing and simple documents. The word processor has taken a backseat to today's desktop and notebook computers.

Typewriters. Most typewriters use correctable film ribbons that pass through the spool only one time. However, if the typewriter uses a cotton or silk ribbon that becomes lighter with use, be sure to change the ribbon before the resulting type impression becomes too light. The typewriter keys need to be cleaned frequently in typewriters that use a cotton ribbon. Typewriters, too, are all but archaic compared with the versatility of the computer.

Copiers. When a typewriter is used to compose a document, a copier may be used for making any necessary copies of the original. Here, too, maintain the copier so that copies are crisp and clear. The toner must be changed when needed and can be expensive. Multiple copies of documents are usually made on a copier rather than printed from the computer.

Scanners. Occasionally, documents are scanned and sent by email. Scanners provide high resolution and can produce images of written text and photos. Scanners are often used to create images so that older documents can be stored, much like the microfiche systems of the past.

1. A word processor is used mainly for:
   a. composing documents
   b. letter writing and simple documents
   c. producing images of written text and photos
   d. making copies of original documents

2. Documents may be scanned and sent by email using a
   a. computer
   b. copier
   c. scanner
   d. word processor

3. A difference between typing and word processing is
   a. a typewriter is more suitable for home and office use
   b. a typewriter is used in homes and the word processor is used for business
   c. a word processor has functions beyond the capabilities of the typewriter
   d. a typewriter is easier to use

4. Scanning eliminates
   a. making carbon copies of the document
   b. making copies of the document
   c. the need for paper files
   d. printing the document

5. Saving and reusing documents is
   a. an advantage of the typewriter
   b. an advantage of making copies
   c. a disadvantage of word processing
   d. an advantage of computers

6. Adding graphics to documents
   a. is possible with computers
   b. are possible with word processing
   c. are always done with a typewriter
   d. are done more easily by retyping

7. Toner is used in
   a. computers
   b. word processors
   c. copiers
   d. scanners

8. Multiple copies of a document should be made on a
   a. scanner
   b. computer
   c. copier
   d. typewriter

9. Spreadsheets can be added to a document when using a
   a. scanner
   b. computer
   c. copier
   d. typewriter

10. Which of the following is the oldest piece of equipment?
    a. computer
    b. word processor
    c. typewriter
    d. copier

LEARNING HOW TO ANSWER SHORT-ANSWER QUESTIONS

Short-answer questions ask you to fill in the blank. When you decide on an answer, check to see that your answer fits into the sentence in both meaning and grammar.

Example 15–2

Directions: Read the following excerpt adapted from a health care textbook (Purtilo, p. 15). Then answer the short-answer questions based on the excerpt. Read the explanation of the answers.

Ethicists have as their primary career activity the work of ethics. At one level they analyze issues. They help to clarify the moral character, values, duties, and other aspects of morality in specific situations. (Medical ethicists or health care ethicists specialize in areas of health care). At another level they work to resolve issues. They work as consultants in the design of ethical policies and practices. But ethics is not the work of ethicists or ethics committees only. Ethics is the work of everybody.

There are two major areas of ethical analysis, metaethics and normative ethics.

1. People who study ethics are called _____.

2. The two major areas of work for ethicists are to _____ issues and _____ issues.

3. Ethics is part of the life of _____.

The answer to question 1 is *ethicists*. If you answered *philosopher* or *theologian*, you would have given an answer that was partly correct.

The answer to question 2 is *analyze* and resolve. This answer can be found in the first paragraph of the passage.

The answer to question 3 is *everybody*. If you answered *philosopher* or *theologian*, you again would have been only partly correct.

EXERCISE 15–2

Directions: Read the following excerpt from a health care text (Purtilo, pp. 73-74). Answer the short-answer questions based on the selection. Use the strategies you learned for answering short-answer questions.

PAYING ATTENTION TO OUTCOMES

Partially because of some of the criticisms of deontology, *teleologic theories* emerged, placing the focus on the ends brought about and the consequences of actions. The most important teleologic theory for our consideration of health care ethics is *utilitarianism.* This word takes its root from the idea of *utility* or usefulness.

In utilitarianism an act is right if it helps to bring about the best balance of benefits over burdens, in other words, the best consequences overall. This approach was developed first by two English philosophers, Jeremy Bentham (1748-1832) and John Stuart Mill (1806-1873). Note that they are roughly contemporaries of Kant. In fact, they were vigorous opponents of Kant's position.

Consider Pam Faden's question about why she is having so much difficulty. How should one decide what Ron Rachels or Metsui Hasagawa should do? From a utilitarian point of view, first you must consider what several different courses of action could accomplish. You might say, "The goal is to treat Pam Faden in such a way that everyone else will be able to have the same type of care she gets," or "The goal is to be able to live with my own conscience." If both these goals can be attained by taking one, single course of action, it should be taken. If this is not possible, the course of action you believe will bring about the best consequences overall should take priority.

One important task of this approach is to distinguish alternate paths of action and then predict as accurately as possible the consequences of each path. As you can begin to see, this approach also has some inherent challenges. How can anyone predict all the potential consequences of an act? Moreover, doesn't this approach ignore that at least sometimes humans do think in terms of their duties, rights, and responsibilties to one another?

1. Teleological theories are concerned with _____.

2. The most important teleological theory for consideration in health care ethics is

   _____.

3. Name two philosophers who developed a utilitarian approach: _____

   and _____.

4. A _____ point of view considers the end, or goal.

5. The word utility means _____.

6. In utilitarianism, an act is right if it brings about the best _____ overall.

7. List two goals of health professionals considering Pam Faden's case from a utilitarian point of view.

   a. _____

   b. _____

8. Name two philosophers who disagreed with Kant's position: _____ and

   _____.

9. If all goals cannot be reached by one action, which consequences take priority?

   _____ .

10. Teleological ethics ignores the fact that sometimes humans do think in terms of their _____ _____ and _____ to one another.

LEARNING HOW TO ANSWER MATCHING QUETIONS

When answering matching questions, link answers from one column to explanations in another column. Keep track of the answers you have already used. In this way you monitor your progress. Matching questions are often used to link words with definitions or to connect cause-effect relationships.

Example 15–3

Directions: Read the following excerpt from a health care textbook (Purtilo, p. 8). Then answer the *matching* questions based on the excerpt. Read the explanation of the answers. Match the *causes* in column A with the *effects* in column B. There is one extra answer.

Duties is a language that has evolved to describe actions in response to claims on you that are either self-imposed or imposed by others. Moral duties describe certain *actions* required of you if you are to play your part in preventing harm and building a society in which individuals can thrive. *Moral character* or *virtue* is a language used to describe *traits* and *dispositions* or attitudes that are needed to be able to trust each other and to provide for human flourishing in times of stress, such as compassion, courage, honesty, faithfulness, respectfulness, humility, and other ways of being in the world that we want to be able to count on. These traits taken together and exercised regularly make up what we mean when we say a person is "of high moral character."

A	**B**
___ 1. A commitment to acting in certain ways	a. Apology
___ 2. Feeling that you wronged someone	b. Obligation
___ 3. Make a promise	c. Commitment to a group
	d. Try to keep it

To answer these questions correctly you would have to understand the relationship between the cause (why) and the result (what) in each column.

The answers are

<u>b</u> 1.

<u>a</u> 2.

<u>d</u> 3.

A commitment to acting in a certain way leads to a feeling of obligation. The feeling that you wronged someone leads to an apology. If you make a promise, the result is that you try to keep it. A commitment to a group is the extra answer. It is not the result of the causes given.

EXERCISE 15-3

Directions: Read the following excerpt from *The Language of Medicine*, by Chabner. Answer the matching questions based on the selection. Use the strategies you learned for answering the matching questions. Match the explanations in column B to the terms in column A.

Fracture Traumatic breaking of a bone.

A **closed fracture** means that a bone is broken but there is no open wound in the skin, whereas an **open (compound) fracture** means a bone is broken and a fragment of bone protrudes through an open wound in the skin. A **pathological fracture** is caused by disease of the bone such as tumor or infection, making it weak. **Crepitus** is the crackling sound produced when ends of bones rub each other or rub against roughened cartilage.

Some examples of fractures are the following:

Colles fracture – occurs near the wrist joint at the lower end of the radius.

comminuted fracture – bone is splintered or crushed into several pieces. A simple fracture means that a bone breaks in only one place and is therefore not comminuted.

compression fracture – bone is compressed; often occurs in vertebrae.

greenstick fracture – bone is partially broken; it breaks on one surface and only bends on the other, as when a green stick breaks; occurs in children.

impacted fracture – fracture in which one fragment is driven firmly into the other.

Treatment of fractures involves **reduction**, which is restoration of the bone to its normal position. A **closed reduction** is manipulative reduction without a surgical incision; in an **open reduction,** an incision is made into the fracture site. A **cast** (solid mold of the body part) is applied to fractures to immobilize the injured bone. In some cases, metal plates, screws, rods, or pins (internal fixation) are utilized to stablize and maintain an open reduction.

COLUMN 1		COLUMN II
1. greenstick fracture	_____	A. fracture of the lower end of the radius at the wrist
2. closed fracture	_____	
3. comminuted fracture	_____	B. break in bone with wound in the skin
4. compound (open) fracture	_____	C. one side of the bone is fractured; the other side is bent
5. Colles fracture	_____	
6. cast	_____	D. bone is put in proper place without incision of skin
7. open reduction	_____	
8. closed reduction	_____	E. mold of the bone applied to fractures to immobilize the injured bone
9. impacted fracture	_____	
10. compression fracture	_____	F. bone is broken by pressure from another bone; often in vertebrae, bone is partially flattened.
		G. bone is splintered or crushed
		H. bone is put in proper place after incision through the skin

I. bone is broken and one side of the fracture is wedged into the other

J. break in the bone without an open skin wound

LEARNING HOW TO ANSWER TRUE-FALSE QUESTIONS

When answering the true-false questions,

- Pay attention to the part of the question that makes it either true or false.
- Pay close attention to detail before you choose your answer.
- Remember that the whole statement has to be correct for the answer choice to be true.
- If part of the statement is incorrect, the answer is false.

Example 15–4

Directions: Read the following excerpt from EMT *Prehospital Care*, by Henry and Stapleton, p. 308; then answer the true-false questions based on the excerpt. Read the explanation of the answers.

Radio communication requires special skills and techniques to ensure the clear and accurate transfer of information. Because many units may be competing for time in the same airspace, radio communications are more concise than conversations over the telephone.

When making initial radio contact, you should never interrupt another radio transmission. Most systems use unit codes or names to identify each caller to the dispatcher. In your initial contact, identify yourself by announcing your code to the dispatcher. After acknowledgement by the dispatcher, you can proceed with your brief transmission. You should speak in a normal (or monotone) voice with the microphone a few inches away from your mouth. The tendency is to speak too loudly or quickly when providing patient care in a serious situation; doing so may garble your message. Unlike telephone conversations, radio allows only one person to speak at a time. While you speak, you must hold down a button, which prevents you from being interrupted by the person to whom you are speaking. This is another reason to keep your messages brief.

At the end of each exchange between you and the other party, give a signal, such as saying "over," to indicate that you are finished speaking and are ready to receive the other person's response. Likewise, you should wait until you hear the same code ("over") from the other party before you press the button to speak again. When speaking on the radio, keep principles of good radio communication in mind.

1. _____ Communications over the radio should be long and clear.

2. _____ It is acceptable to interrupt another radio transmission. You should identify yourself by announcing your code to the dispatcher.

3. _____ Radio transmissions are only one way at a time.

4. _____ You should not speak in a monotone voice.

5. _____ The term "over" indicates that you are finished speaking.

The answer to question 1 is "false" because part of the answer is incorrect. Conversations over the radio should be short, not long. The answer to question 2 is "false." The first sentence of paragraph 2 states that you should never do this. Be aware of the word not when reading. It changes the meaning of the sentence. The answer to questions 3 is true. The information is found in the second paragraph. The answer to question 4 is false. In this case the word **not** in the statement changes the information in the last sentence of the passage, and makes the answer "false." The answer to question 5 is "true." The information can be found in the last paragraph.

EXERCISE 15–4

Directions: Read the following excerpt from a health care text (Henry and Stapleton, p. 57). Answer the true-false questions based on the selection. Use the strategies you learned for answering true-false questions.

ABANDONMENT

As an EMT who is part of an EMS system, you assume the responsibility of providing care to an ill or injured patient from the time you arrive on the scene until you transfer the patient to the care of hospital personnel. **Abandonment** is a legal term that describes a situation in which an EMT or other health professional discontinues a patient-provider relationship without giving the patient time or opportunity to obtain continuation of care at the same level or higher. This includes circumstances in which an EMT on the scene leaves a patient who is in need of emergency care and transportation to a hospital or when an EMT prematurely discontinues care.

For a case of abandonment to hold up in court, complainants must first establish that they were owed a duty and that the duty was breached.

Charges of abandonment are also possible if a patient who refused care was incompetent, such as a child or an adult with an altered mental status, yet was left at the scene. If the EMT suspects that a patient who refuses care is not capable of making a reasonable judgment, he or she should make every attempt to transport that patient to the hospital. If the patient adamantly refuses, you should secure the aid of family, medical control, and/or police officers. In some instances, transporting the patient against his or her will may be appropriate and necessary. If administrative or legal advice is available in such circumstances, you should avail yourself of this help.

_____ 1. Abandonment is a form of litigation.
_____ 2. Only EMTs are subject to abandonment litigation.
_____ 3. Charges of abandonment is possible in cases in which a person who refuses care is incompetent.
_____ 4. It is never appropriate to take the patient against his will.
_____ 5. As an EMT you are responsible for patient care from the time you arrive on the scene until one week after you transfer the patient to hospital care.
_____ 6. An example of an incompetent patient would be a child or adult with an altered mental state.
_____ 7. Care that is prematurely discontinued is not a case of abandonment.
_____ 8. If an EMT leaves the patient on the scene in need of emergency care, the EMT can be charged with abandonment.
_____ 9. If the patient cannot make a reasonable judgment, every attempt should be made to transport the patient to the hospital.
_____ 10. If an incompetent patient refuses care, the EMT should not contact the family.

EXERCISE 15–5

Directions: Read the following excerpt from a health care textbook (Henry and Stapleton, pp. 29-30). Study the material and then answer the objective test questions based on the material.

SPREAD OF COMMUNICABLE DISEASES

Infectious agents spread from a source to a host. A *source* of infection may be a person, an insect, an object, or another substance that carries or is contaminated by an infectious agent. A *reservoir* is a source in which infectious agents can live and multiply, such as a sewer.

After a microorganism infects a susceptible person or host, it can multiply until symptoms of the disease appear. The time between *contact* with an infectious agent and the onset of signs and symptoms of the disease is called the **incubation period**. During the incubation period the host may or may not be infectious to others, depending on the particular infection. The period during which a person can transmit an infectious disease to others is called the **communicable period**. The communicable period may be before, during, and even after the occurrence of symptoms of a particular disease. A **carrier** is a person who shows no signs of the disease yet harbors an infectious organism and may be a source of the infection to others.

Exposure is a term used to signify coming in contact with, but not necessarily being infected by, a disease-causing agent. The type of exposure (how you were exposed) and the degree of exposure (how much you were exposed to the agent) can vary greatly and these are factors in determining whether a person is more likely to become ill. For example, the type of exposure necessary to transmit disease varies for each infectious agent. Some diseases, such as measles, can be transmitted through the air (airborne). Other diseases, such as human immunodeficiency (HIV), the virus that causes AIDS, are not spread through airborne contact or casual contact but require close contact, such as blood to blood or sexual intercourse for transmission.

In terms of degree of exposure, a critical mass of infectious agent usually is required to cause infection. And although that critical number varies among agents, the simple concept is the greater the number of microorganisms transmitted to the host, the more significant the exposure. For example, a person who receives a transfusion of contaminated blood has a greater exposure than a person who experiences a needle stick with a contaminated needle from the same source.

Some organisms have a greater infective potential than others. For example, hepatitis B virus is much more likely than HIV to cause infection if a health care worker gets a needle stick from a needle contaminated with the virus.

Health care workers are exposed to patients with infectious conditions as part of their work. Infectious diseases that are spread by health care workers or within a health care setting are called *nosocomial infections.*

Not everyone who is exposed to a source of infection becomes sick. Understanding which factors and conditions of an exposure can lead to actual infection is part of infection control. These factors include the following:

- Mode of transmission
- Type and duration of contact
- Host susceptibility
- Whether appropriate precautions were used

Part I. After reading this selection, fill in the blanks.

1. Infectious agents spread from a source to a _____.

2. A _____ is a source in which infectious agents can live and multiply.

3. A person who shows no sign of the disease yet harbors an infectious organism and may be a source of infection to others is a _____.

4. The time between contact with an infectious agent and the onset of signs and symptoms is called the _____.

5. _____ is a term used to signify one's coming in contact with, but not necessarily being infected by, a disease-causing agent.

Part II. Match the letters in column B with the numbers in column A.

A	**B**
____ 1. HIV	a. airborne disease
____ 2. communicable period	b. infectious diseases that are spread by health care workers
____ 3. measles	c. the greater the number of organisms transmitted to the host, the more significant the exposure
____ 4. nosocomial infections	d. time period in which one can transmit an infectious disease
____ 5. critical mass of infection	e. AIDS virus

Part III. Answer the multiple-choice questions based on the passage you have read.

1. A source of infection may be
   a. a person
   b. an insect
   c. an object
   d. all of the above
2. A person who shows no sign of the disease, yet harbors an infection
   a. source
   b. host
   c. carrier
   d. infectious agent
3. A patient hospitalized with hepatitis B:
   a. source
   b. resevoir
   c. carrier
   d. host
4. A sewer, for example
   a. source
   b. resevoir
   c. carrier
   d. host
5. The time between contact with an infectious agent and the onset of signs and symptoms is called
   a. the communicable period
   b. casual contact
   c. the incubation period
   d. lack of exposure

Part IV. Read the following statements. In the space provided write "T" if the statement is true or "F" if the statement is false.

1. AIDS is the virus that causes HIV._____

2. During the incubation period, the host is never infectious to others. _____

3. The communicable period may be before, during, and even after the symptoms of a particular disease occur. _____

4. Everyone who is exposed to a source of infection becomes sick. _____

5. The type of exposure necessary to transmit disease is the same for each infectious agent._____

EXERCISE 15–6

Directions: Read the following excerpt from a health care textbook (Henry and Stapleton, pp. 868-869). Create you own objective test based on the selection. Create five short-answers, five matching, five multiple-choice, and five true-false questions.

ACUTE RADIATION SYNDROME

High doses of <u>radiation</u> absorbed over a short period, such as minutes to hours, can cause signs and symptoms of acute radiation syndrome. This syndrome results from damage to the bone marrow, gastrointestinal tract, central nervous system, and cardiovascular system as the dosage increases. For example, at an exposure of 50 rem, patients may have no visible effects, but a small percentage of persons who have been exposed may show a depression of white blood cells and platelets on blood testing. Physical signs and symptoms may first appear at a dose of 100 rem, with nausea and vomiting occurring in a small percentage of exposed persons. At 200 rem, most patients show signs of nausea and vomiting with more profound depression of the bone marrow. At 400 rem, about 50% of the exposed individuals die within weeks. An exposure of 600 rem can result in a near 100% death rate if there is no medical intervention.

At doses of 1000 rem, <u>gastrointestinal</u> complications begin to appear as nausea, vomiting, and diarrhea of immediate onset. At doses of 3000 rem there are additional irreversible cardiovascular effects resulting in irreversible <u>hypotension</u> and a central nervous system syndrome with rapid onset of drowsiness, uncoordination, and convulsions.

Emergency Medical Care of Victims of Radiation

The main focus on emergency care is treatment of associated injuries, removal from further exposure, and decontamination.

Once a patient has been irradiated, there is little to be done at the scene. Illness usually follows hours to days later. The main focus is to limit continued exposure and treat associated injuries.

The contaminated victim requires attention to minimize the risk of internal contamination and incorporation. Through decontamination, the potential for internal contamination and secondary spread is reduced. If internal contamination has occurred, then treatment to minimize the chance of incorporation should be considered as soon as possible.

Personal Protection and Factors Affecting Severity of Exposure

The major factors used by rescuers to limit exposure are *time*, *distance*, and *shielding*.

The severity of radiation exposure is affected by the strength of the radioactive source, the type of radiation, the duration of exposure, the area of the body exposed, the distance from the radioactive source, the amount of shielding between the source and the victim, and the age and condition of the patient.

Duration of Exposure

The shorter the time spent in a radiation field, the less radiation the body absorbs. For example, if the exposure rate is 100 R/hour, 15 minutes in the area may result in absorption of 25 R. Rescue workers can reduce individual exposure by sharing the time spent in the danger zone to perform a rescue.

Distance from the Source

The greater the distance from the source of radiation, the less the radiation dose absorbed. If the source of radiation emanates from a single point, radioactivity falls inversely with the *square of the distance*. Thus if one doubles the distance away from the source, the absorbed dose falls off by a factor of 4. And if the distance is tripled, it falls off by a factor of 9.

If radiation sources are scattered, this inverse square rule does not apply. However, radiation exposure is decreased significantly by increasing the distance from the material.

Learning Strategies for Taking the Essay Test

In an essay test, students are expected to state the main ideas and to support those general statements with details. Also, students should be able to draw conclusions from ideas presented. Clear, simple, organized writing, as well as content, often counts toward your grade.

Before Writing Your Answer

- Read the entire test carefully.
- Pay close attention to the directions.
- Look at the point value of each question. You should spend more time on a question worth 30 points than on one worth 10 points.
- Read the questions carefully.
- Understand the question. Are you asked to list, explain, classify, contrast, or sequence information?
- Allow time for reading questions, thinking about, and organizing your answers.
- Arrange your thoughts. Write an outline.

While Writing Your Answer

- State the main idea in a clear topic sentence.
- Support main ideas with relevant details.

After Writing Your Answer

- Read all your answers.
- Check to see that you have answered the questions that were asked.
- Make sure that you have answered all parts of each question.
- Make necessary changes in content, mechanics, and organization.
- Use an editing checklist to help you revise your essay.

Following is an example of an editing checklist:

CONTENT   YES   NO

Are the ideas developed?   ____   ____
Is the presentation logical?   ____   ____
Are the examples appropriate?   ____   ____

MECHANICS

Did you check your choice of words?   ____   ____
Did you improve the sentence structure?   ____   ____
Did you make sure your use of punctuation is correct? ____   ____

ORGANIZATION

Does your essay contain an introduction?   ____   ____
a body with supporting evidence?   ____   ____
a conclusion?   ____   ____

Example 15–5

Directions: Read the following excerpt from *Ethical Dimensions in the Health Professions* by Purtilo, p. 205. Review the sample essay question and answer based on the selection.

Genetic information has enhanced the questions about the possibilities that individuals have a right not to know about information that could be harmful, shameful, or embarrassing about themselves and that they would choose not to know.

Suppose that Meg's daughters are identical twins. If one is tested and found to have the gene composition that gives her a high probability for the development of breast and ovarian cancer, and she decides to take the drastic measure of a prophylactic radical mastectomy before the appearance of cancer, her sister (who has the identical genetic makeup as her twin) who did not want to know inevitably *will* know that she has the gene.

The two sisters meet with Helen and discuss their conflict. Twin A says she will consider it abandonment if she is not tested and allowed to make this choice. Twin B says that she will be betrayed if, having been offered the opportunity and refused, Twin A is given the opportunity for testing then takes steps that will in fact reveal the status to Twin B. Is there any moral claim on the genetic team not to proceed with the genetic testing of Twin A?

The possibility of "the right not to know" certainly supports the idea that the professional ought not to force informaiton on a client, compromising her psychological defenses and well-being. In our current story, however, the psychological well-being of one twin (A) appears in direct conflict with the other (B), and the resolution between them probably cannot be solved satisfactorily by the health professionals refusing to offer testing, counseling, and treatment to Twin A.

In summary, genetic information is especially powerful because of its ability to involve whole kinships. The extra precautions of care that physicians, geneticists, and genetic counselors use in disclosing genetic information provide useful cautions for all health professionals in the disclosure of any sensitive information.

Do you think that you should have the right to not know genetic information? Why? Why not?

SAMPLE ANSWER

NOTE: In the following paragraph the first sentence introduces the topic of the paragraph; the next three sentences provide the supporting details; and the final sentence supplies the conclusions.

Individuals have the right to *not* know certain medical information. Prenatal testing provides information about the genetic health of a fetus as well as its sex. Some parents choose to wait until the birth of the child to find out if they are having a boy or a girl. This decision to "not know" does not affect the baby to be. Therefore there are times when an individual can exercise his/her right to not know medical information without harming others.

EXERCISE 15-7

Directions: Read the following excerpt from the Purtilo health care textbook, pp. 201-202. Answer the following essay question based on the selection.

PLACEBOS: A SPECIAL CASE OF INFORMATION DISCLOSURE

The issue of *placebo* use has received some attention from psychiatrists and ethicist, but most of the literature on placebos has been directed toward physicians. Little research has been done concerning the role of other health professionals and the use of placebo medications and procedures and yet nurses and pharmacists, in particular, play a direct and essential part in this particular form of deception in health care practice. To think clearly about the ethical problems that may arise in such a situation it is important to understand the physician's role in prescribing a placebo and some of the history and psychology of the placebo response.

Placebo comes from the Latin word meaning "I shall please." It can be defined as any therapeutic procedure (or component of one) that is given for a condition on which it has no known pharmacologic effect. A pure placebo is a preparation of an inert substance that is not known to have any pharmacological effect. An impure placebo is an active drug given for its psychological effect even though it has no known effect on the disorder in question, such as an antibiotic for a common cold or other viral infection. Administering the latter type of placebo carries the risk of real side effects, as well as the interpersonal and professional risks we will discuss in regard to pure placebos.

Physicians rarely give pure placebos, such as sugar pills or saline injections, but when they do, serious ethical issues need to be considered. One important aspect of the practice of giving placebos is what is called the placebo effect. Virtually all treatments (and also some diagnostic studies) have positive effects for some patients over and above the specific effects of their pharmacological mechanisms. Beecher published a classic study in 1955 showing that placebos are effective in treating pain in 35% of patients, regardless of the source of pain or clinical condition of the patient. Later studies have done little to alter these percentages. Modem neuropharmacology research has discovered that the brain produces its own chemicals which can act as analgesics and relaxants. These chemicals, called endorphins, seem to work better for some people than for others, which may explain scientifically why some people react to placebo and others do not. A common error made by health professionals has been the assumption that a symptom (e.g., pain) successfully treated by a placebo is therefore not real or is "only psychological."

The placebo effect may be partly responsible for the success of ancient remedies given by shamans or medicine men. Some of these remedies contained pharmacologically active agents, but others did not, and much of the healer's work consisted of rituals and symbols. That the medicine men often were successful is a tribute to the power of the therapeutic partnership.

Modern examples of the placebo effect are the effects of suggestion in decreasing stomach acid in patients with ulcers, alleviating bronchospasm in asthma, and decreasing blood pressure. The phenomenon of the placebo effect is widespread and powerful enough so that no research trials of new medications or even surgical procedures are considered truly rigorous unless the element of suggestion has been effectively eliminated, as in randomized, double-blind clinical trials.

Some ethicists and others oppose the use of placebos in health care because they see it as an example of deception or outright lying. We have considered the problem of lying to patients in regard to the disclosure of situations that have serious consequences for the patient.

Question: Weigh the positive effects against the possible negative effects of administering placebos to patients. Then decide whether you think it is unethical to use placebo medications in patient care.

Strategy 5: Evaluate Test Results

Once your test paper is returned, don't just look at your score and throw away the paper. Look at what you know. Look at what you still need to learn. Go back to your notes and text to correct all errors. If you still need help, schedule a conference with your study partner, study group, and/or your instructor. Save all test papers. Use these tests to review for your final exam.

REVIEWING STRATEGIES FOR IMPROVING TEST SCORES

TO LEARN	USE THIS STRATEGY
To plan ahead	Apply time management skills.
To keep up with assignments	Be an active reader.
	Use active listening and effective note taking strategies.
To study and learn material	Review class notes and text, summaries and outlines, and underlined material.
	Organize information into categories.
	Review vocabulary.
	Pay attention to illustrations and formulas.
	Use mnemonics to improve your memory.
	Monitor your learning.
	Discover your best study method.
	Design practice tests.
To take the test successfully	Learn strategies for taking objective tests.
	Learn strategies for taking essay tests.
To evaluate test results	Look at what you know.
	Look at what you still need to learn.

UNIT V

READING SELECTIONS

In Unit V, Reading Selections, you will apply all the strategies you learned in Units I through IV. Each reading selection is an excerpt from a text in the allied health fields. The exercises based on the readings are designed to give you practice in the reading, writing, mathematics, and study strategies that you learned in the other units. Unit V can be used throughout the semester or as a final unit once Chapters 1 to 15 are completed. When you have completed Unit V, you will be prepared to successfully read and study from your textbooks in the allied health fields.

Reading Selection
1

PREVIEW QUESTION

- What are the reasons you chose to enter the allied health care field? What do you expect from your new career?

VOCABULARY

Directions: Locate five words that are new to you in this reading. Write the meaning of each of these words in the space provided.

_____

_____

_____

_____

_____

_____

_____

_____

_____

A career as a medical assistant is challenging and offers variety, job satisfaction, opportunity for service, fair financial reward, and possibility for advancement. It is open to both men and women.

ADVANTAGES

The trained medical assistant is equipped with a flexible, adaptable career. The skills acquired by the medical assistant are valuable, and employment is readily available anywhere in the world that medicine is practiced. Individuals working in the medical assisting field do not have a **mandatory** retirement age. Many medical assistants pursue their careers far beyond the usual retirement age, because physicians realize the value of the experienced, mature employee. This career attracts the nontraditional student who may be older than the average postsecondary

From Young AP, Kennedy DB: *Kinn's the medical assistant: an applied learning approach,* ed 9, St Louis, 2003, Saunders, pp 43-44.

student by a decade or more. Although many older students feel intimidated by the classroom, they normally have excellent experiences in school and become top in their class. Medical assisting is more than suitable for the student just exiting high school, who may plan on continuing his or her education and plans to use medical assisting as a viable income during further studies.

The practice of medicine has changed dramatically in the past several decades. Increasing costs have created a trend away from hospital-based treatment and moved toward the delivery of care in physicians' offices and in outpatient ambulatory clinics. Although physicians have employed medical assistants in their practices for many years, computerization and technologic advances have created more opportunities for formally trained medical assistants and their responsibilities have similarly increased. Clearly defined educational requirements have been determined by the nation's two certification organizations. These requirements have resulted in improvement of the quality and accessibility of medical assistant training, and have produced a healthy respect for medical assistants, who are considered a part of the allied health field.

Employment for medical assistants is abundant. There were 329,000 jobs held by medical assistants in the United States in 2000, and 60% of those were in physicians' offices. Career opportunities abound in public health facilities, hospitals, laboratories, medical schools, research centers, voluntary health agencies, and medical firms of all kinds. Jobs may also be available with federal agencies such as the Department of Veterans Affairs, the U.S. Public Health Service, and armed forces clinics or hospitals.

Most medical assistants derive a high degree of satisfaction from their work. Job turnover among medical assistants is surprisingly low; some medical assistants begin working with a physician when the practice is opened and stay until the physician's retirement. Most physicians have learned that "bargain help" is often the most expensive.

Medical assistants are compensated in various ways, some hourly and some by salary. The earnings vary from place to place. Overall, medical assistants can expect a healthy return on their investment in training, experience, and skills. Most physicians realize that a good medical assistant is worth a higher-than-average wage, and a medical assistant with formal training often is compensated on a higher scale than one with no training. The *Occupational Outlook Handbook*, a Department of Labor publication, keeps statistics on the average salaries for many different career fields, including medical assisting. This information can be accessed at http://stats.bls.gov/ocohome.htm. More information on salaries may be obtained by monitoring the local help-wanted advertisements and by checking online job offer information on sites such as Yahoo! Careers. It is important to determine a realistic entering salary. Often graduates in many fields expect to make a much higher salary than is reasonable right after graduation.

The medical field often offers very good **benefits** to employees. Usually, the larger the organization, the better the benefits and **perks**. Most employers offer a health insurance plan or managed care plan to their employees. Often a moderate life insurance program is included, and dental insurance is always a valuable benefit. There are companies that have **profit sharing** plans and **stock options**. Some organizations give their employees access to credit unions, and many have discount options to local businesses, such as at a uniform shop. Remember that benefits and perks should be included when considering a certain job. Many medical assistants may choose to work for less money if the benefits and the opportunities for advancement are good. One should also consider driving time, holidays, paid parking, sick days, vacation days, and facilities when choosing a job. Do the co-workers seem to enjoy each other and get along? Is the physician friendly or more "stand-offish" and cold? All of these should be weighed carefully before making the final decision as to which position to accept. It is a truism that "money is a by-product of services rendered." Nowhere is this more accurate than in the medical field. When the patients are served well, the medical assistant becomes more and more valuable to the employer and is compensated accordingly.

WRITING

Directions: Answer the following question based on the reading selection. Remember to use the following writing strategies:

- Organize ideas
- Write the first draft
- Revise, edit, and proofread to write the final draft

What personal qualities must an individual have to become a successful medical assistant?

COMPREHENSION QUESTIONS

Directions: Answer the multiple-choice questions based on the selection. Use the strategies you learned for answering multiple-choice questions.

1. At 65 years old, or retirement age, a medical assistant
   a. must retire
   b. needs to take a complete medical examination
   c. can continue working
   d. must renew state certification

2. A position as a medical assistant is
   a. available only in the United States and Canada
   b. not available in Africa and Asia
   c. only available in the city where you trained
   d. available anywhere that medicine is practiced

3. A medical assistant's work can be in
   a. a laboratory
   b. a physician's office
   c. a medical firm
   d. all of the above

4. The salaries for medical assistants are
   a. the same throughout the country
   b. the same throughout the world
   c. different in rural and urban areas
   d. different depending on your training

5. A medical assistant may check statistics on average salaries by using all of the below except
   a. this text
   b. local help wanted advertisements
   c. Yahoo! Careers
   d. the Occupational Outlook Handbook

6. The duties of a medical assistant will
   a. vary from office to office
   b. be uniform from office to office
   c. be independent of the doctor's habits
   d. always be clerical

7. Benefits and perks
   a. are always part of a salary package
   b. always include profit sharing
   c. usually increase with the size of the organization
   d. should not be considered when evaluating a job offer

8. The United States has how many certification organizations for medical assistants?
   a. one
   b. two
   c. three
   d. four

9. Employment for medical assistants is
   a. only in hospitals
   b. not well paid
   c. abundant
   d. not available after the usual retirement age

10. There is a low turnover among medical assistants because
    a. there are few job openings
    b. medical assistants are afraid of losing their retirement benefits
    c. medical assistants are fearful of getting poor references
    d. many enjoy working with their physicians

WORD PROBLEM

Directions: Use the strategies you learned for solving word problems to answer this question:

A medical assistant living in New York City makes $35,000 annually. How much does he make per month? A medical assistant in a farming town in Mississippi makes $9,000 less. How much does she make annually? How much does she make monthly?

Reading Selection
2

PREVIEW QUESTIONS
- What questions can you create from the boldface headings?

VOCABULARY

Directions: Locate five words that are new to you in this reading. Write the meaning of each of these words in the space provided.

_____

_____

_____

_____

_____

_____

_____

_____

_____

_____

SOFTWARE

All computers require an *operating system* that assists in managing the different hardware devices in the computer. The system manages the keyboard and the mouse input, video and sound output, and data storage devices such as the *hard drive*. The various compact disk drives and floppy drives are also managed by the operating system. The majority of computers today use a Microsoft Windows 95 or 98 operating system, although a few computers still use MS-DOS (Microsoft Disk Operating System). Other operating systems available are Microsoft Windows NT (New Technology), 2000, or ME; Macintosh OS (Apple Computer Operating Systems); and LINUX. Today, most operating systems are capable of multitasking, a characteristic that means that they can have multiple programs running simultaneously. The *graphical user interface* (GUI) screens made popular by the Windows operating system let the user switch between multiple programs without having to close out of each program.

From Diehl MO: *Diehl and Fordney's medical transcription: techniques and procedures*, ed 5, St Louis, 2002, Saunders, pp 30-33.

Additionally, a computer typically requires some kind of *work processing software* to enable the transcriptionist to key in, format, and edit dictation. Word processing software can be as basic as the DOS-based WordPerfect 5.1 or as complex as Microsoft Word. Most Windows-based word processors have features that make repetitive tasks easier and quicker. Some features include automatic text insertion and formatting, document templates or boiler-plating, macro creation, spell checking, word and line counting, and thesaurus research. Many more add-on software packages are available that can enhance the functions as well. The most common targeted for the medical industry are *word expanders*, which allow the MT to create abbreviations that expand into words of any length as well as complete sentences or paragraphs. Also available are medical and pharmaceutical dictionaries and spell checkers with tens of thousands of medical words that can be added to the standard word processor's dictionary or accessed in the spell-checking function.

SPEED TYPING SYSTEMS

Word Expansion Programs

The most popular method of quickly inputting data into a computer is to use a word expansion program. These programs run in the "background" of your word processing program and "watch" for certain predefined abbreviations, sometimes called short forms, from the keyboard. Whenever the abbreviations are typed, the program automatically expands the characters or numbers into a predefined word, phrase, or complete sentence. This feature comes in handy when keying in very long words or frequently used phrases, a common requirement in medical transcription. These programs are designed to help the production transcriptionist increase productivity while reducing the number of keystrokes entered. These programs also help improve accuracy by enabling the medical transcriptionist to create distinct abbreviations for words that frequently present spelling or fingering problems. For example, if you often type "yu" for "you," you simply teach your computer to turn "yu" into "you." If you spell it correctly, you still get "you."

Macros

A *macro* is typically a small program or set of instructions that the word processors uses to complete repetitive tasks. A popular task that macros are typically used for is to take an existing paragraph or a complete document and perform a "find and replace" function to insert text at a certain location in a document. Macros can be set up to be accessed by a key sequence or a mouse click. Generally, a key-sequence macro is called a "keyboard macro," because the macro is activated by pressing a certain set of keys on the keyboard. Frequently used macros include symbols that you like to use that are not represented on your keyboard. For example, the degree symbol hides until a command key and a set of numbers on the keypad are depressed. You make a macro that produces the symbol with a simple command of your own making, maybe "ds." If you forget your command, you can easily access your entry list or vocabulary to check on it.

Template

Templates are used to generate formats that have the same structure every time they are created. Once set up correctly, a template can be set with a "read-only" attribute so it cannot be changed. With this feature, new documents can be generated from the template without modifying the original one accidentally. Templates are very popular for formats in which the header, paragraph headings, and footer are always the same and the text body is the only part that changes.

ONLINE INFORMATION PROCESSING SYSTEMS

In medium and large companies, many users may require access to shared information on large information networks (Figure V-1). The development of LANs, WANs, and the Internet has enabled users to share information, peripherals, e-mail, optical character readers, and data

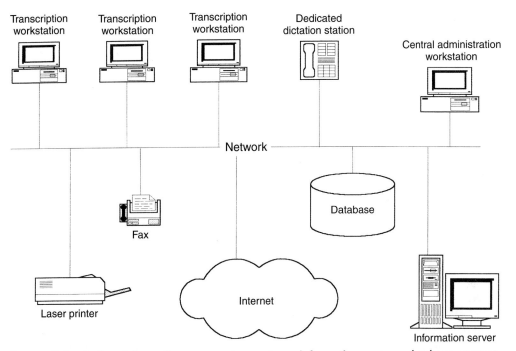

FIGURE V-1 Online information processing system: information server, database storage, connection to the Internet, online fax system, shared printers, several transcription workstations, dedicated dictation station, and a central administration workstation.

storage devices. A network typically contains one or more large, more powerful computers called *servers* connected to several smaller computers called *workstations*. Online information processing systems take advantage of this network technology by using the servers to store large amounts of information in databases that are then accessed by the users on the workstations. The information can be quite extensive, such as large databases containing electronic patient records, drug indexes, insurance information, typed and scanned documents, and digital voice files. Because all the information data can be stored on the server, managing the information from one central location is much easier. The central administrator can distribute the work and produce reports as well as archive and back up data. When dictation is recorded into the system, the dictated material can be associated with a patient record, type of dictation, and the author's name; the dictation is subsequently assigned to a transcriptionist. When the transcriptionist accesses the digital voice file from the system at the click of a mouse, all of the important information about the patient and the dictator is instantly available with the dictation. The dictated voice files can be flagged for priority so the transcriptionist can prioritize the work efficiently. Once the voice file is transcribed, it can be sent to a printer or filed for later retrieval. Two popular online information processing systems in the medical industry are Dictaphone's Enterprise Express Voice System and Lanier's Cquence.

DATA STORAGE
Hard Disk Drive

The hard drisk drive, usually located inside the computer case, is the component that stores large amounts of data for quick retrieval. The *hard disk* gets its name from the physical characteristics of the disk inside the drive unit. These disks, or "platters," are very rigid and can withstand extremely high spin rates. Because the hard disk spins so fast, in order to avoid disk crashes, it is important to keep the disk very stable while it is turned on. The hard disk drive is not portable from one computer to another, so the computer must be part of a network for multiple computers to be able to access the data on the hard disk.

Compact Disk–Read-Only Memory

A *compact disk–read-only memory* (CD-ROM) is much more portable than a hard drive, but CD-ROMs cannot hold as much data. CD-ROMs are used mainly for distributing software, because once a CD-ROM is "written to," it cannot be changed. A CD-ROM is also more durable than a hard drive, because the CD-ROM is not a magnetic medium like the hard drive. A CD-ROM is made of a metallic sheet sandwiched by two pieces of plastic. The data are stored on the metallic sheet in the form of very small pits that are "read" by a laser. Some variations of the CD-ROM exist, such as the *compact disk–rewriteable* (CD-RW), which can be changed after it has been written to, but CD-RWs require a special drive unit.

Floppy Disk

A magnetic media *diskette* is a 3.5-inch, thin, circular piece of magnetically coated plastic that is contained in a protective cover to shield its surface from contamination by dust and fingerprints. Storage capacity is determined by whether the diskette is single or dual sided and single or double tracked.

Data Backups

Hard disks can "crash" and floppy disks can be easily damaged, so making backups of your data files is very important. There are several ways to make a backup file. If you are backing up floppy disks, make copies of the floppy disks and store the copies in a separate location. If you are backing up your hard disk, use a tape backup or a CD-RW to back up the data. Test your backup at least once a month to make sure the data can still be read from the media. You do not even want to guess at your dismay if you need to restore data from a backup and find the backup is unreadable. If the system does not automatically back up the data, then you should perform manual backups on a daily basis.

Because you will have important information stored on computer disks, it is vital to take care of them. The information is magnetically recorded. Therefore, any magnetic or electromagnetic field can scramble or destroy data recorded onto a disk. Your telephone, printer, and video terminal contain magnetic fields, so do not place a disk on top of this equipment. Disks should be properly stored in boxes. The container should be kept away from extreme heat (100° F or above) and out of direct sunlight, because the information could be destroyed or the disk could melt. Never attach rubberbands to disks, because these could bend or damage the disks.

Always label each disk before filing it in the storage box. Do not stack labels on a disk. Too many labels could cause an imbalance in the weight of the surface of the disk and may make it difficult for the computer head to read the data. Keep disks clean and out of the way of possible spills or stains. Never drink, eat, or smoke around the computer area. If a disk case must be cleaned, use a damp cloth to wipe it off.

Printer

The two most popular printer types are ink jet and laser. The ink-jet printers make print by shooting a very fine stream of ink at the paper. Typically, these have the capability of printing in color; however, they are slower than laser printers and do not have a very high degree of print quality. Laser printers use a laser beam to magnetically charge certain areas of a light-sensitive drum. Once the drum has been charged, a powderlike substance or toner is applied to the drum. The paper is then passed over the drum to transfer the toner to the paper. The toner is bonded to the paper by a heat process. Laser printers produce much higher printer quality but of course are also much more expensive than are ink-jet printers both to operate and to purchase. Paper output from a printer is called *hard copy* and can vary greatly in quality. Paper quality is measured in weight. Heavier weight paper tends to be thicker and more expensive than lower weight paper.

In many transcription departments, printing may be done off site. It is common for documents to print in another room in the building or across town or to be transmitted via modem to a hospital floor for accessibility. Therefore, it cannot be overemphasized that you must read data on the screen while transcribing, because you may not get another opportunity.

Laser printers are fitted with toner cartridges. Some companies sell recycled, refilled cartridges, which are less expensive than new cartridges. However, check for high-quality refill toner, and ask whether the company replaces the drum in each cartridge before the cartridge is refilled. This practice guarantees crisp clean printouts.

Data Communications and Modems

The word *modem* is an acronym for **mod**ulator **dem**odulator unit. Modems are used to communicate from one computer to another computer within a facility, to transmit data to another computer in a remote area, or to send data to the Internet over standard telephone lines. In today's world of high-speed Internet access, it is important to use an equally high-speed modem such as Integrated Services Digital Network (ISDN), Digital Subscriber Line (DSL), and cable modems. Regardless of which data communications medium you use, however, data security is important. When transmitted over any communication medium, data are susceptible to *hacking* by someone other than the sending or receiving parties. The key to data security is to make it as difficult as possible for the hacker or eavesdropper to do anything with the data once he or she obtains the file. Therefore, a cryptosystem should be part of your Internet transfer of documents. The basic idea behind data encryption is for the sender to encrypt the data files by using a key, which is typically made up of a string of data bits (1s and 0s). The key at the receiving end is some value that allows the message to be decrypted and read. Note that the lengths of keys are described in terms of *bits* in cryptosystems. The longer the key, the more difficult it is to break an encrypted message. Many good cryptosystems are available for document protection.

Some transcription services offer telecommunication via modem. Then they can transmit correspondence or reports to an office, a clinic, or a hospital facility many miles away. Documents transmitted in this way can be revised and edited at the receiving office before they are printed out into hard copy.

WRITING

Directions: Answer the following question based on the reading selection. Remember to use the following writing strategies:

- Organize ideas
- Write the first draft
- Revise, edit, and proofread to write the final draft

What role do you see computers playing in the health care professions?

COMPREHENSION QUESTIONS

Directions: Answer the true and false questions based on the selection. Use the strategies you learned for answering true and false questions.

1. MS DOS stands for Microsoft digital operating system.   T____F____
2. A macro is used for frequently used symbols not on the keyboard.   T____F____
3. Word expansion programs watch for predefined abbreviations.   T____F____

4. Windows let you see various programs at one time.   T____F____
5. Smaller computers on a network are called servers.   T____F____
6. Hard disk drives are portable from one computer to   T____F____
   another.
7. A computer modem relies on a telephone.   T____F____
8. A cryptosystem should be avoided when transferring   T____F____
   documents by the Internet.
9. You should test your backup system at least once a year. T____F____
10. Laser printers are fitted with toner cartridges.   T____F____

WORD PROBLEM

Directions: Use the strategies you learned for solving word problems to answer this question:

Howell General Hospital has 18 cassette-changer central recorders. Each of these recorders holds 15 cassettes. How many cassettes can be used in total? Nine allied health workers have been trained to use these central recorders. How many cassettes can each worker use at one time?

Reading Selection
3

VOCABULARY

Directions: Locate five words that are new to you in this reading. Write the meaning of each of these words in the space provided.

_____

_____

_____

_____

_____

_____

_____

_____

_____

_____

_____

_____

THE SKIN CONSISTS OF THE EPIDERMIS AND DERMIS

Skin consists of two main layers: an outer **epidermis** (ep'-ih-**der'**-mus) and an inner **dermis** (**der'**-mus). Beneath the skin is an underlying **subcutaneous** (sub'-koo-**tay'**-nee-us) **layer** (Figure V-2).

The Epidermis Continuously Replaces Itself

Over most parts of the body, the epidermis is only about as thick as a page of this book, yet it consists of several sublayers. The epidermis consists of stratified squamous epithelial tissue. The outer cells of the epidermis continuously wear off and are immediately replaced by new cells. New epidermal cells are constantly produced in the deepest sublayer of the epidermis. These cells mature as they are pushed toward the outer surface by newer cells beneath. As they move toward the body surface, epidermal cells manufacture **keratin** (**ker'**-ah-tin)—a tough water-proofing protein that gives the skin mechanical strength and flexibility. As epidermal cells

From Solomon EP: *Introduction to human anatomy and physiology,* ed 2, St Louis, 2003, Saunders, pp 41-42.

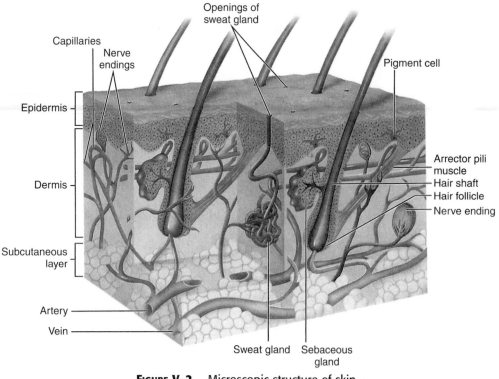

FIGURE V–2 Microscopic structure of skin.

move through the outer sublayer of epidermis, they die. The cells at the surface of the skin resemble dead scales. They are closely packed together and serve as a waterproof protective covering for the body.

The Dermis Provides Strength and Elasticity

The dermis is the thick layer of skin beneath the epidermis (see Figure V-2). Dermis consists of dense connective tissue composed mainly of collagen fibers. Collagen is largely responsible for the mechanical strength of the skin. It also permits the skin to stretch and then return to its normal form again. Blood vessels and nerves, which are generally absent in the epidermis, are found throughout the dermis. Specialized skin structures such as hair follicles and glands are found in the dermis. They develop from cells of the epidermis that push down into the dermis.

The upper portion of the dermis has many small, fingerlike extensions, called **dermal papillae** (pah-**pil'**-ee), that project into the epidermal tissue. Extensive networks of capillaries in the papillae deliver oxygen and nutrients to the cells of the epidermis and also function in temperature regulation. The patterns of ridges and grooves visible on the skin of the soles and palms (including the fingertips) reflect the arrangement of the dermal elevations beneath. Unique to each individual, these patterns provide the fingerprints so useful to law-enforcement officials. They also serve as friction ridges that help us hold onto the objects we grasp.

The Subcutaneous Layer Attaches the Skin to Underlying Tissues

The subcutaneous layer beneath the dermis is also known as the **superficial fascia** (**fash'**-ee-ah). This layer consists of loose connective tissue, usually containing a lot of adipose (fat) tissue. The subcutaneous layer attaches the skin to the muscles and other tissues beneath. This thick fatty layer helps protect underlying organs from mechanical shock. It also insulates the body, thus conserving heat. Fat stored within the adipose tissue can be mobilized and used as an energy source when adequate food is not available. Distribution of fat in the subcutaneous layer is largely responsible for characteristic male and female body shapes.

WRITING

Directions: Answer the following question based on the reading selection. Remember to use the following writing strategies:

- Organize ideas
- Write the first draft
- Revise, edit, and proofread to write the final draft

What is the overall importance of the skin for humans?

COMPREHENSION QUESTIONS

Directions: Answer the matching questions based on the selection. Use the strategies you learned for answering matching questions.

SKIN LAYER	FUNCTION	
A. Epidermis	Attaches skin to muscle	1. ____
B. Dermis	Protects organs from mechanical shock	2. ____
C. Superficial fascia	Blood vessel and nerves found here	3. ____
	Serves as a waterproof cover	4. ____
	Allows the skin to stretch	5. ____
	Insulates the body	6. ____
	Conserves heat	7. ____
	Capillaries deliver oxygen to cells	8. ____
	Cells are pushed to outer surface by newer cells	9. ____
	Helps with temperature regulation	10. ____

WORD PROBLEM

Directions: Use the strategies you learned for solving word problems to answer this question.

All individuals have their unique set of fingerprints, or visible ridges and grooves, on the tips of their fingers. Detective Hogwood is investigating a crime scene. Luckily, he has been able to find the fingerprints of the perpetrator. However, they are not complete. Nevertheless, he runs them through the computer looking for a partial match. Out of the 206,000 prints registered in the computer, 20% of them are potential matches. How many people does this represent?

Reading Selection
4

PREVIEW QUESTION
- What systems of the body does this selection discuss?
- What you already know about the systems?

VOCABULARY

Directions: Locate five words which are new to you in this reading. Write the meaning of each of these words in the space provided.

_____

_____

_____

_____

_____

_____

_____

_____

_____

THE SKELETAL SYSTEM
The Skeletal System

The bones of the skeleton (Figure V-3) are divided into axial and appendicular portions. The axial portion consists of the skull (cranial and facial bones), vertebral column, and thorax (sternum and ribs). The appendicular portion consists of the shoulder girdle, pelvic (hip) girdle, and bones of the upper (arm) and lower (leg) extremities. There are 80 bones in the axial portion and 126 bones in the appendicular portion of the skeleton. The skeletal system provides the framework of the body, protects vital organs, and works with the muscular system to produce movement. Blood cells are produced within the red marrow of the bones. Orthopedics is the medical specialty that studies the skeletal system and associated structures.

DIAGNOSTIC TESTS	DISORDERS
Alkaline phosphatase (ALP)	Arthritis
Calcium	Bursitis

From Flynn JC: *Procedures in phlebotomy,* ed 3, St Louis, 2005, Saunders, pp 16-24.

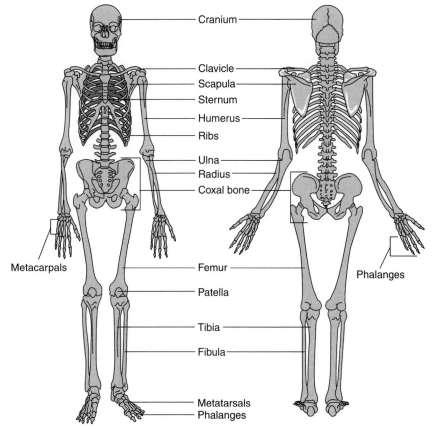

FIGURE V-3   Anterior and posterior views of the skeletal system.

DIAGNOSTIC TESTS

Complete blood cell count (CBC)

Erythrocyte sedimentation rate (ESR)

Synovial fluid analysis

Uric acid

DISORDERS

Gout

Osteoporosis

Tumors

The Muscular System

Muscle tissue is differentiated by its appearance, location, and function. There are three types of muscle tissue:

1. **Smooth muscle** tissue **(visceral)** is located in the walls of blood vessels and hollow organs such as the stomach. This tissue looks smooth or nonstriated because it lacks alternating light- and dark-colored bands. It is involuntary muscle tissue, which means it needs stimulation from hormones or nerve transmitter substances to function.
2. **Cardiac muscle** tissue forms most of the heart. This tissue is striated because it has varying bands and is involuntary. The contraction of this muscle is usually not under the body's conscious control and is responsible for the heart's ability to beat.
3. **Skeletal muscle** tissue primarily attaches itself to the bones and helps to move the skeleton. It is striated and voluntary because it can be made to contract and relax with conscious control.

The body is composed of more than 700 muscles (Figure V-4). Muscles need a source of energy to function. For example, glucose from the blood enters the contracting muscle. Oxygen releases the energy from the glucose, and it is converted to the energy form **adenosine**

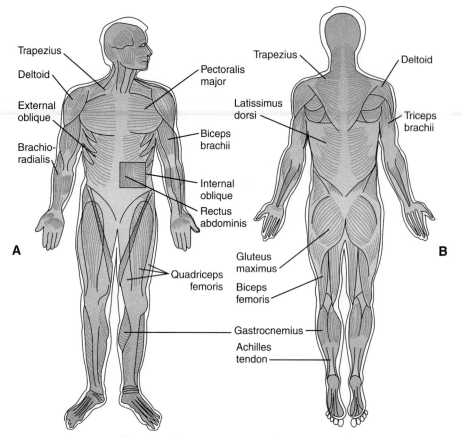

FIGURE V-4 The muscular system. **A,** Anterior view. **B,** Posterior view.

triphosphate (ATP). Calcium then interacts with the contractile filaments within the muscle cells. Oxygen is not always required for muscle function; however, if this **anaerobic** process continues for an extended period, **lactic acid** accumulates in the blood and muscle tissue. This buildup soon causes muscle fatigue. As skeletal muscle contracts to work, heat is generated. Much of the heat is used to maintain normal body temperature. For example, a football player helps to keep his body warm by actively participating in the sport even in very cold weather. Myology is the study of muscles.

DIAGNOSTIC TESTS

Creatine kinase (CK) and Isoenzymes

Lactate dehydrogenase (LD or LDH)

Lactic acid

Myoglobin

DISORDERS

Muscular dystrophy

Myalgia

Tendinitis

THE NERVOUS SYSTEM

The purpose of the nervous system is to detect changes, known as stimuli, from both internal and external environments. It then analyzes the information and coordinates an appropriate response. Nerve cells, or **neurons**, conduct impulses from the receptors in the body to and within the central nervous system (CNS). The body also uses chemicals called neurotransmitters to carry impulses between neurons. A common neurotransmitter is acetylcholine. The junction between two neurons is called a synapse.

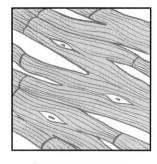

Cardiac muscle fibers

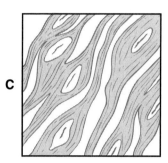

Smooth muscle (visceral)

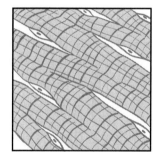

Skeletal muscle

FIGURE V–4, cont'd.   C, Types of tissues.

The nervous system is divided into two sections (Figure V-5). The CNS consists of the brain and spinal cord. The peripheral nervous system (PNS) consists of all nervous tissue outside the CNS. The PNS is further divided into the somatic nervous system (SNS) and the autonomic nervous system (ANS) (Figure V-6). The SNS conveys information from the head, body wall, and extremities to the CNS. The CNS then sends impulses to the skeletal muscle. The ANS conveys information from the viscera to the CNS. The CNS then sends impulses to the stomach, cardiac muscle, and glands.

The ANS is further divided into two systems: the sympathetic and the parasympathetic. The sympathetic system stimulates or excites the organ to start activity. This is known as the "fight or flight" response. The parasympathetic system decreases or inhibits activity to restore and maintain balance. Neurology is the medical specialty that studies the nervous system.

The sensory organs, a component of the nervous system, contain many receptor cells that can detect stimuli. The receptors may be widely distributed or localized in the sense organs within the body. The sense organs include the eye, ear, tongue, and nose. They are responsible for vision, hearing and equilibrium, taste, and smell, respectively. General receptors detect

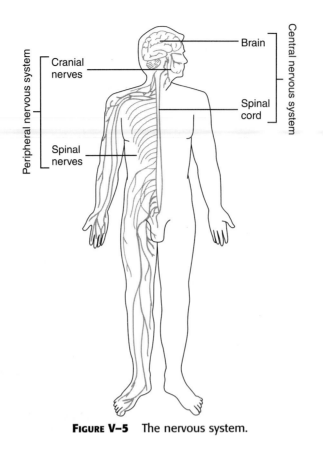

Peripheral nervous system

Cranial nerves

Spinal nerves

Brain

Spinal cord

Central nervous system

FIGURE V–5 The nervous system.

touch, pain, pressure, and temperature. The medical specialties that diagnose abnormalities within this system include ophthalmology (eyes) and otolaryngology (ears, nose, and throat).

DIAGNOSTIC TESTS	**DISORDERS**
Acetylcholine receptor antibody	Amyotrophic lateral sclerosis (ALS)
Cerebral spinal fluid (CSF) analysis	Epilepsy
Cholinesterase	Meningitis
Drug levels	Multiple sclerosis (MS)
Rapid *Streptococcus* screen	Parkinson's disease
RAST tests (allergy screens)	Shingles

THE ENDOCRINE SYSTEM

The body contains two types of glands that secrete substances that affect other cells: exocrine and endocrine. Exocrine glands secrete substances into ducts that are then carried to organs or body cavities or outside the body. Sweat glands are an example of this type. The remainder of the discussion will be devoted to endocrine glands, which constitute the endocrine system. Endocrine glands secrete their substances or **hormones** into the space around the secretory cells. Examples of these glands include the **pituitary**, which is regulated by the **hypothalamus** in the brain; the **thyroid**, which is located below the **larynx** or voice box; and the **adrenals**, which lie superior to each of the kidneys. Figure V-7 shows the major endocrine glands.

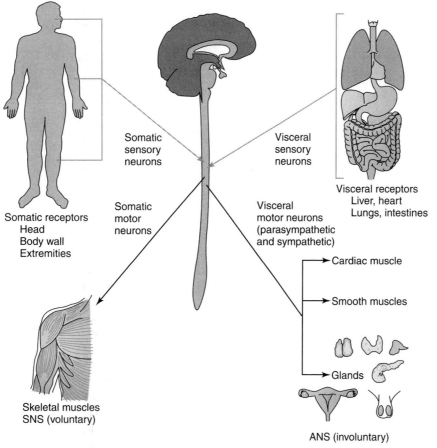

FIGURE V-6   The somatic nervous system and autonomic nervous system.

Hormones are very powerful substances. They regulate metabolism and energy production, contraction of muscles, growth, and aspects of the immune system. They also help to maintain homeostasis within the body and play an important role in the reproductive cycle from its initial stages of gamete production through delivery of the newborn infant. Prolactin, insulin, and oxytocin are just a few of the many hormones secreted in the human body. Endocrinology is the study of the endocrine system.

DIAGNOSTIC TESTS

Adrenocorticotropic hormone (ACTH)

Aldosterone

Antidiuretic hormone (ADH)

Catecholamines

Cortisol

Glucose tolerance tests

Insulin

Testosterone

Thyroid function studies

   (T3, T4, thyroid stimulating hormone [TSH])

DISORDERS

Cushing's syndrome

Diabetes insipidus

Diabetes mellitus

Dwarfism

Hyperthyroidism

Hypothyroidism

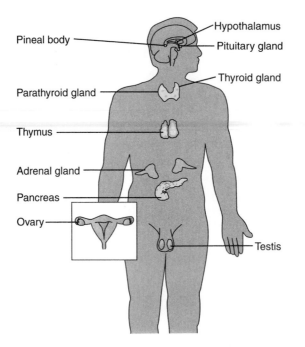

FIGURE V–7 The endocrine system.

THE CARDIOVASCULAR SYSTEM

All cells within the body must be constantly supplied with nutrients and oxygen. The circulatory system (Figure V-8) is responsible for this function. It also removes waste products and carbon dioxide by transporting them to the proper sites for disposal. Additionally, it helps to control body temperature. The circulatory system consists of the heart, which pumps blood through blood vessels. The lymphatic vessels return **lymph**, which is very similar to interstitial fluid, to the blood. This makes the lymphatic vessels an auxiliary part of the circulatory system.

WRITING

Directions: Answer the following question based on the reading selection. Remember to use the following writing strategies:

- Organize ideas
- Write the first draft
- Revise, edit, and proofread to write the final draft

What are the similarities and differences between the cardiovascular and lymphatic systems?

COMPREHENSION QUESTIONS

Directions: Answer the short-answer questions based on the selection. Use the strategies you learned for answering short-answer questions.

1. The three types of muscles are smooth, _____ and skeletal muscles.
2. Approximately how many muscles move the skeletal system?_____

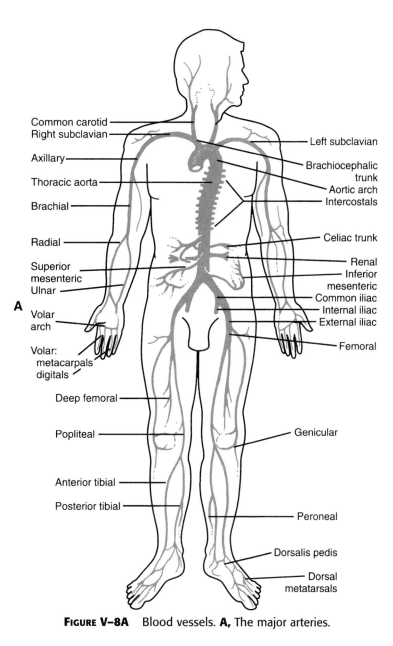

Common carotid
Right subclavian
Axillary
Thoracic aorta
Brachial
Radial
Superior
mesenteric
Ulnar
A
Volar
arch
Volar:
metacarpals
digitals
Deep femoral
Popliteal
Anterior tibial
Posterior tibial

Left subclavian
Brachiocephalic
trunk
Aortic arch
Intercostals
Celiac trunk
Renal
Inferior
mesenteric
Common iliac
Internal iliac
External iliac
Femoral
Genicular
Peroneal
Dorsalis pedis
Dorsal
metatarsals

FIGURE V–8A   Blood vessels. **A,** The major arteries.

Continued.

3. CNS stands for the _____.

4. The _____ controls information from the viscera to the CNS.

5. The bones of the skeleton are divided into _____ and _____ portions.

6. Which cells carry impulses between neurons?_____

7. Which system consists of the heart and blood vessels? _____

8. Prolactin and insulin are examples of _____.

9. Blood carries away _____ and _____.

10. Body heat is generated by _____.

infer that even now the cat is not fully domesticated because it can revert to total self-sufficiency. The time from ancient Egypt to the present may represent as few as 4000 generations with a constant infusion of genes from uncontrolled populations. Only the small group of purebred cats had true selective breeding, and these are mainly for physical features. The first recorded planned feline breeding did not occur until 999 AD at the Japanese Imperial Palace. It soon became fashionable in that country to control cat matings and environments. With cats under tight control mice devastated the silkworm industry, so by 1602 Japanese cats were again released from these controls.

Although the cat fell from favor and met with mass extermination in Europe, selective breeding was of course not practiced. Even with the Crusaders helping its return to favor, the atmosphere was one of tolerance rather than full acceptance. Historically, then, it took many years before the cat achieved a position in which selective breeding could help develop the behavioral characteristics desired in a domesticated animal.

CURRENT STATUS OF THE FELID
Cat Population Statistics

In recent years there has been a dramatic increase in the number of cats, especially registered cats, in the United States, partly because of their adaptability to apartments and small homes. Exact population figures vary greatly and are inaccurate because of the wild population, but it has been estimated that the cat population numbers from 23,100,000 to 61,000,000. In the United States 23% of households have at least one cat. Sixty-six percent of cat owners have only one cat, but associated figures estimate 1.4 to 2.2 cats for each house having cats, or 1 cat in every 3.2 single-family dwelling units. Of this cat population less than 80% are seen annually by veterinarians.

The modern cat's lifestyle tends to fall into one of four categories: (1) feral, independent "wildlife," totally ignored by people; (2) feral and interdependent free-roaming or unowned with dependence to humans limited to food; (3) domesticated, interdependent, and free-roaming or loosely owned, such as abandoned pets; and (4) domesticated household pets. Of this owned group, only 14% of the cats are purebred, compared with 61% of owned dogs. The population is also relatively young, with 11% younger than 1 year, 49% being 1 to 6 years, 27% being 7 to 12 years, and 10% older than 12 years.

The number of stray cats has been estimated at between 2% and 28% of the known population. Whereas 415 humans are born every hour in the United States, 100 to 2000 kittens are born per hour. The significance of this is that at least 30,000 cats must die per day just to maintain a stable population. At the end of a 1-year period 18% to 30% of cats are no longer in their original home. After 3 years two thirds are no longer in their first home.

An excess population comprises those animals that are available and adoptable but for which no home can be found. Each year as many as 20% of a city's pet population may pass through its animal shelter. An estimated 4 to 9 million cats die each year in these shelters. Of all cats euthanized in shelters, 18% to 33% die because of behavior problems. At least 28% of cats relinquished to animal shelters are there because of behavior problems. The top four problems cited include housesoiling, problems between pets, aggression toward humans, and destructive behaviors. Interestingly, the presence of at least one other pet in the home dramatically increases the likelihood of relinquishment for behavior problems to approximately 70%, a trend that has been especially true if a new pet was added during the preceding year.

The surplus cat population is related to the cat's reproductive efficiency and cat owners' attitudes. Although most of the U.S. population believes that something should be done about pet overpopulation, most cat owners claim their own litters "just happen." Half believe controlling reproduction is the pet owner's responsibility, but a lot of ignorance remains about the necessity of neutering. People who relinquish cats to animal shelters are significantly more likely to believe a female should have a litter before being neutered and to be ignorant about the estrous cycle compared with cat owners who keep their cat. They also are more likely to believe that cats exhibit behaviors for "spite," to not understand normal play behaviors, and to feel the number of cats in a home does not relate to the incidence of problems.

In 7 years one female cat can be responsible for the birth of up to 781,250 kittens. In 7.9% of cat-owning households at least one litter of kittens is born during the year and most of those are unplanned. By the time a queen is 3 years old, 74.4% will have had at least one litter, and many of the females that do have an ovariohysterectomy have already had kittens. The highest cat densities are found in the same areas that have the highest densities of people—a source of food. The presence of these cats indicates that there is a niche that will support that approximate number of cats, so migration and reproduction help replace any permanent losses. Removal of individual cats increases population turnover but does not significantly alter the total number of cats. The large stray feline population may be reflected in another statistic: Only 38% of male cats are castrated and 31% of females are spayed, although local differences are reported.

Worldwide cat ownership is increasing, often in parallel to trends in the United States. In several European countries, the numbers for cats increased so much that they now outnumber dogs, as did the percentage of homes owning cats.

Cat Owner Categorization

In addition to surviving a varied history, the cat has survived many types of owners. Cat owners have been classified in several ways by different researchers, but they tend to be categories for those who have a weak attachment and those who have a strong one. The classification "low involvement owner" is applied to 59% of the 14,645,000 cat-owning households in one study of pet owners. Another study called this group "pet dispassionates" and suggested it comprised 41% of pet owners. These individuals devote little time to the care or company of the cat and seem to enjoy having a cat around more than really interacting with it. The animal may be a companion for someone else in the household. This lack of involvement with the pet is reflected in trauma statistics. Of 126 cats (89 males, 37 females) reported injured over slightly more than a year's period, 16.3% were hit by a car, 14.7% were involved in animal interaction, and 39.5% received injuries from causes unknown to the owner. Although the average age for the general population is 3 years, that of the neutered cat is 3 to 5 years longer, and that of the traumatized cat is only 1.3 years. This is despite the average life span for a cat being 12 years, with ages of 20 years or older not uncommon. The current longevity record is 36 years. One study of roadkills indicated that most were kittens or young adults. Because of these low involvement owners, cat populations for the most part still fulfill the criteria of random mating.

A subcategory of the low-involvement group might include owners described as the "pet-for-child people." This group consists of 29% of owners. Here the pet is considered to belong to a child; the adult is not highly committed to the animal but usually ends up being the primary caregiver.

The second classification of cat owners, those with a strong attachment, has been subdivided. "Quality or status conscious owners" represent 21% of all cat owners. The pet is an expression of how this owner views himself or herself and reflects his or her good taste, as would other material possessions. These owners feel that the cat depends on them for love, affection, and care, and as a result, the animal is well groomed and only reluctantly left alone.

"High involvement owners" compose the second subdivision of the strong-attachment category. These owners have also been called "pet owners" and make up 20% to 30% of pet owners. Unlike owners in the other two categories, these individuals rely on the cat to supply love and affection or to serve as an emotional crutch, such as child substitute. Attachments to the cat are frequently described as those to a human family member, friend, or child. These people feel the cat enjoys humans, feed it specially prepared foods, have photographs of the pet, take it on vacation, and may celebrate the cat's birthday. They estimate spending more than 3 hours a day with the animal, particularly on the weekend. Owners from this group are most likely to bury a deceased pet in a pet cemetery or mausoleum or to leave an estate to their cats. Just this kind of owner made two cats worth $415,000 in 1965 the richest cats in history.

Cat owners with a strong attachment to their pets are often in the middle and upper socioeconomic levels and will spend billions of dollars each year on their pets. These individuals have a higher percentage of neutered cats and a preference for lighter-colored cats.

WRITING

Directions: Answer the following question based on the reading selection. Remember to use the following writing strategies:

- Organize ideas
- Write the first draft
- Revise, edit, and proofread to write the final draft

If you were a cat owner, would you be a low-involvement owner or a high-involvement owner? Explain.

COMPREHENSION QUESTIONS

Directions: Answer the multiple-choice questions based on the selection. Use the strategies you learned for answering multiple-choice questions.

1. The cat was brought into the house from the wild for
   a. work reasons
   b. companionship reasons
   c. religious reasons
   d. utilitarian reasons

2. Some experts believe that the cat is not fully domesticated because the cat
   a. is totally self-sufficient
   b. is capable of biting
   c. does not get along well with dogs
   d. basically does not like humans

3. In the 1600s the cat fell out of favor in
   a. Japan
   b. Europe
   c. Egypt
   d. United States

4. The population increase of cats in the United States is due to
   a. the decline of dogs
   b. the increase in the rodent population
   c. their ability to be independent
   d. their ability to live in small dwellings

5. Most cat owners are
   a. low-involvement owners
   b. high-involvement owners
   c. part high- and part low-involvement owners
   d. neither low- nor high-involvement owners

6. The majority of cats killed on the road are
   a. elderly cats
   b. partially blind cats
   c. kittens and young adults
   d. nursing mothers of young kittens

7. The type of owner who would celebrate a cat's birthday is
   a. the low-involvement owner
   b. the high-involvement owner
   c. always childless and lonely
   d. none of the above

8. The number of cats that see a veterinarian range between
   a. 3 and 13 million
   b. 15 million and 17 million
   c. 20 and 60 million
   d. undetermined

9. Cat ownership worldwide is
   a. stabilizing
   b. unknown
   c. decreasing
   d. increasing

10. You can conclude from this selection that the writer
    a. favors cats
    b. dislikes cats
    c. neither likes nor dislikes cats
    d. cannot determine

WORD PROBLEM

Directions: Use the strategies you learned for solving word problems to answer this question.

Assume that the pet cat population is 56 million and that the stray cat population represents 10% of the pet cat population. How many cats are stray cats?

Reading Selection
6

PREVIEW QUESTION
- What are the six members of the dental healthcare team?

VOCABULARY

Directions: Locate five words that are new to you in this reading. Write the meaning of each of these words in the space provided.

_____

_____

_____

_____

_____

_____

_____

_____

_____

_____

ROLES AND RESPONSIBILITIES OF DENTAL HEALTHCARE TEAM MEMBERS

Dentist or Dental Specialist
- Is legally responsible for the care of the patient.
- Assesses the patient's oral health needs as related to physical and emotional well-being.
- Uses up-to-date diagnostic skills.
- Uses current techniques and skills in all aspects of patient care.
- Provides legally required supervision for dental auxiliaries.

Clinical Dental Assistant (Chairside Assistant, Circulating Assistant)
- Seats and prepares patients.
- Maintains and prepares treatment rooms and instruments.
- Assists dentist at chairside during patient treatment.

From Bird DL, Robinson DS: *Torres and Ehrlich modern dental assisting,* ed 8, St Louis, 2005, Saunders, p 2.

- Prepares and delivers dental materials.
- Provides postoperative patient instructions.
- Oversees infection-control programs.
- Performs radiographic procedures.
- Performs basic laboratory procedures (e.g., pouring impressions to create diagnostic casts).
- Provides assurance and support for the patient.

Expanded-Functions Dental Assistant

- Performs only those intraoral (inside mouth) procedures that are legal in the state in which the EFDA practices.
- Check with your state board of dentistry for a current listing of dental assistant duties.

Dental Hygienist

- Assesses the periodontal status of patients, including measurement of the depth of periodontal pockets and conditions of the oral tissues.
- Performs dental prophylaxis (e.g., removal of plaque from crowns and root surfaces).
- Performs scaling and root-planing procedures.
- Exposes, processes, and evaluates the quality of radiographs.
- Performs additional procedures, such as administration of local anesthetic and administration of nitrous oxide if allowed by the state.

Business Assistant (Administrative Assistant, Secretarial Assistant, Receptionist)

- Greets patients and answers the phone.
- Makes and confirms appointments.
- Manages patient records, payroll, insurance billing, and financial arrangements.
- Ensures that patient privacy measures are in place and followed.
- Oversees patient relations.

Dental Laboratory Technician

- Performs laboratory work only under licensed dentist's prescription.
- Constructs and repairs prosthetic devices (e.g., full and partial dentures).
- Constructs restorations (e.g., crowns, bridges, inlays, veneers).

WRITING

Directions: Answer the following question based on the reading selection. Remember to use the following writing strategies:

- Organize ideas
- Write the first draft
- Revise, edit, and proofread to write the final draft

What type of dental assistant would you choose to be? Give reasons for your choice.

COMPREHENSION QUESTIONS

Directions: Answer the true and false questions based on the selection. Use the strategies you learned for answering true and false questions.

1. The dentist is legally responsible for the care of the patient.　T＿＿ F＿＿

2. Records management is part of an administrative assistant's duties.　T＿＿ F＿＿

3. Making appointments is done by both the dentist and the administrative assistant.　T＿＿ F＿＿

4. The chairside assistant helps with patient seating and preparation.　T＿＿ F＿＿

5. The circulating assistant assesses the periodontal health of the patient.　T＿＿ F＿＿

6. The circulating assistant is responsible for applying topical anesthetics.　T＿＿ F＿＿

7. The dental laboratory technician constructs restorations.　T＿＿ F＿＿

8. "EFDA" stands for "educated for dental assisting."　T＿＿ F＿＿

9. The EFDA performs directly on patients according to state regulations.　T＿＿ F＿＿

10. A clinical dental assistant can perform radiographic procedures.　T＿＿ F＿＿

WORD PROBLEM

Directions: Use the strategies you learned for solving word problems to answer this question.

Ms. Happytooth worked as an administrative assistant in Dr. Fine's office. Ms. Happytooth was responsible for accounts receivable and accounts payable. At the end of the month she had to balance the books. On the accounts payable side, Ms. Happytooth noticed that Dr. Fine received $29,583 in patient fees. On the accounts payable side, she noticed that Dr. Fine paid $16,245 in salaries, $900 in rent, and $1711 in miscellaneous expenses. Did Dr. Fine make a profit for that month, or did he go further into debt? If he made a profit, what was the amount? If he went further into debt, what was the amount?

Reading Selection
7

PREVIEW QUESTION
• What are the organs of the respiratory system?

VOCABULARY

Directions: Locate five words that are new to you in this reading. Write the meaning of each of these words in the space provided.

_____

_____

_____

_____

_____

_____

_____

_____

_____

_____

THE RESPIRATORY SYSTEM
Organs of the Respiratory System
1. Nose
2. Pharynx
3. Larynx
4. Trachea
5. Bronchi
6. Lungs

Division of the Respiratory System

The upper respiratory system refers to the nose, nasal cavities, sinuses, pharynx, and larynx. The lower respiratory system refers to the trachea, bronchi, alveoli, and lungs (Figure V-9).

From LaFleur Brooks M, Gillingham EA: *Health Unit Coordinating*, ed 5, St Louis, 2004, Saunders, pp 536–538.

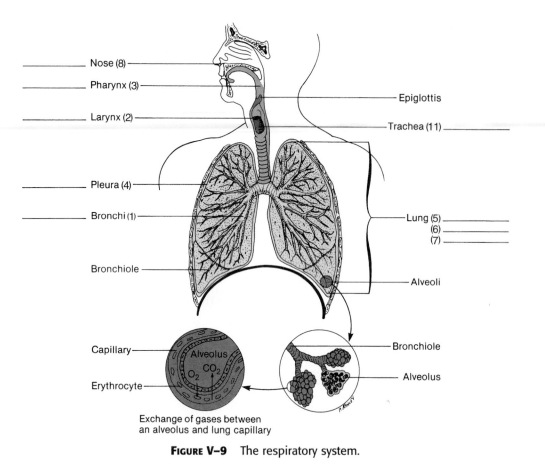

Nose (8)
Pharynx (3)
Larynx (2)
Epiglottis
Trachea (11)
Pleura (4)
Bronchi (1)
Lung (5)
(6)
(7)
Bronchiole
Alveoli
Capillary
Alveolus
CO$_2$
O$_2$
Erythrocyte
Bronchiole
Alveolus

Exchange of gases between
an alveolus and lung capillary

FIGURE V-9   The respiratory system.

Function of the Respiratory System

The function of the respiratory system is to exchange gases. Oxygen is taken into the body and carbon dioxide is removed. This process is referred to as *respiration*. The respiratory system also helps to regulate the acid-base balance and produce vocal sounds.

Respiration

External respiration, or breathing, is the exchange of gases between the lungs and the blood. Oxygen is inhaled into the lungs and passes through the capillary wall into the blood to be carried to the blood cells. Carbon dioxide passes out of the capillary blood to the lungs to be exhaled to the outside environment.

The exchange of gases also takes place within the body between the blood in the capillaries and individual body cells. This is called *internal respiration*. The body cells take on the oxygen from the blood and at the same time give off carbon dioxide to the blood to be transported back to the lungs, where it is exhaled from the body.

The Nose

Air enters the respiratory system through the nose. The nose is divided into a right and left nostril by a partition called the *nasal septum*. The nose prepares the air for the body by (1) warming and moistening the air, (2) removing pathogenic microorganisms, and (3) removing foreign particles, such as dust, from the air. Tiny, hairlike growths in the nose called *cilia* trap and move the foreign particles toward the oustide and away from delicate lung tissue. Particles too large to be handled by the *cilia* produce a sneeze or cough, which forcibly expels the foreign particles.

The Pharynx

Both air and food travel through the *pharynx* (throat). The food passes from the pharynx to the esophagus, while the air passes from the pharynx into the larynx, which is located anterior to the esophagus.

The Larynx

The larynx (voice box) is a tubular structure located below the pharynx. As mentioned earlier, the pharynx is a passageway for both food and air. A flap of cartilage, called the *epiglottis*, automatically covers the larynx during the act of swallowing to prevent the food from passing from the pharynx into the larynx. The larynx contains the vocal cords. As the air is exhaled past the vocal cords, the vibration of the cords produces sounds.

The Trachea

The *trachea* (windpipe), a vertical tube 4 to 5 inches (10 to 12.5 cm) long, extends from the larynx to the bronchi. A series of C-shaped cartilage rings prevents the trachea from collapsing. The function of the trachea is the passage of air.

Bronchi

Behind the heart, close to the center of the chest, the trachea branches into two tubes: one leading to the right lung and the other leading to the left lung. These tubes are called *bronchi* (singular: *bronchus*). The function of the bronchi is the passage of air.

The Lungs

The lungs are cone-shaped organs located in the thoracic cavity. The right lung is the larger of the two and is divided into three lobes. The left lung is divided into two lobes. After the bronchus enters the lung, it divides into smaller tubes and continues to subdivide into even smaller tubes called *bronchioles*. At the end of each bronchiole is a grapelike cluster of air sacs called *alveoli* (singular: *alveolus*). The walls of the alveoli are single celled, which allows for the exchange of gases to take place between the alveoli and the capillaries. The *pleura* is a double sac that surrounds each lung and lines the walls of the thoracic cavity. The *visceral pleura* lines the outer surface of the lungs, whereas the *parietal pleura* covers the chest wall. The small amount of fluid within the sacs allows the lungs to expand and contract without friction.

CONDITIONS OF THE RESPIRATORY SYSTEM
Pneumothorax and Hemothorax

Pneumothorax

Pneumothorax is the collection of air or gas in the pleural cavity, resulting in a collapsed lung, or *atelectasis* (Figure V-10). It may be caused by a chest wound, or it may be a spontaneous collapse due to lung disease. The pleural cavity is airtight, with negative pressure. As air enters the pleural cavity it creates pressure against the lung, causing it to collapse.

Symptoms include sudden sharp chest pain, shortness of breath, cyanosis, and stopping of normal chest movements on the affected side. Treatment ranges from observation and supplemental oxygen for an uncomplicated pneumothorax to a thoracentesis to remove the air or gas from the cavity and a thoracotomy, with the insertion of chest tubes. The tubes are connected to an underwater drainage system with suction and remain in place until air is no longer expelled from the pleural space.

Hemothorax

A *hemothorax* is the collection of blood in the pleural cavity; it is usually caused by chest trauma. Symptoms include chest pain, shortness of breath, respiratory failure, tachycardia, and anxiety. Treatment includes stabilizing the patient, stopping the bleeding, insertion of a chest tube to evacuate the blood and air from the pleural space, and re-expanding the lung.

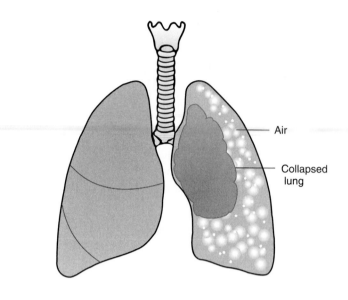

FIGURE V–10 Pneumothorax.

Pulmonary Embolism (PE)

Pulmonary embolism is the most common complication in hospitalized patients. It strikes 6 million adults a year, causing 100,000 deaths. Pulmonary embolism is usually caused by a blood clot that has been dislodged from a leg or pelvic vein, *deep vein thrombosis* (DVT), that blocks a pulmonary artery. Symptoms are cough, dyspnea (difficulty in breathing), chest pain, cyanosis (blue tinge to the skin), tachycardia, and shock. It is difficult to distinguish from pneumonia and myocardial infarction. Chest x-ray, pulmonary arteriography, arterial blood gases, and lung perfusion scans coupled with a lung ventilation scan are used to diagnose pulmonary embolism. Treatment includes thrombolytic, anticoagulant, and oxygen therapy.

WRITING

Directions: Answer the following question based on the reading selection. Remember to use the following writing strategies:

- Organize ideas
- Write the first draft
- Revise, edit, and proofread to write the final draft

What is the passageway of air through the respiratory system? Use sufficient details when writing your answer.

COMPREHENSION QUESTIONS

Directions: Answer the matching questions based on the selection. Use the strategies you learned for answering matching questions.

A. Nose	contains vocal cords	1. _____
B. Pharynx	located behind the heart	2. _____
C. Larynx	cone-shaped organs	3. _____

D. Trachea   nasal septum divides the left and right nostrils   4. _____

E. Bronchi   passage of air   5. _____

F. Lungs   branches into two tubes   6. _____

     where the exchange of gases take place   7. _____

     both air and food travel through this   8. _____

     where airenters the respiratory system   9. _____

     is covered by the epiglottis during swallowing   10. _____

WORD PROBLEM

Directions: Use the strategies you learned for solving word problems to answer this question.

What percentage of people die of pulmonary embolism if 6,000,000 adults are hospitalized with this condition and 100,000 patients die?

Reading Selection
8

PREVIEW QUESTION
- What does figure V-12 describe?

VOCABULARY

Directions: Locate five words that are new to you in this reading. Write the meaning of each of these words in the space provided.

WRITING

Directions: Answer the following question based on the reading selection. Remember to use the following writing strategies:

_____

_____

_____

_____

_____

_____

_____

_____

_____

- Organize ideas
- Write the first draft
- Revise, edit, and proofread to write the final draft

What is the procedure for folding a surgical gown? Write your answer in paragraph form.

Figures V-11 to V-13 are from McCurnin DM, Bassert JM: *Clinical textbook for veterinary technicians*, ed 6, St Louis, 2006, Saunders, pp 693–696.

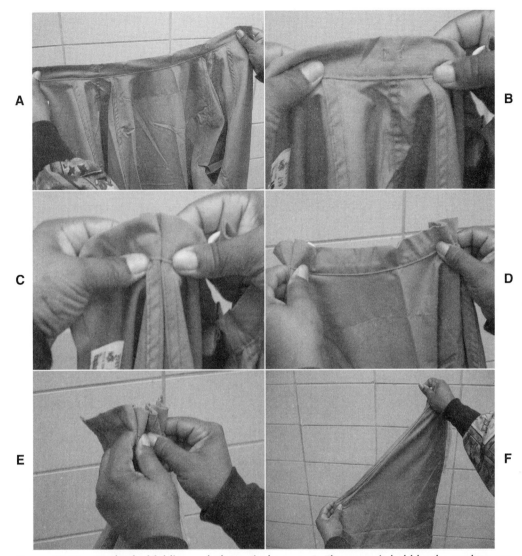

FIGURE V–11   Method of folding a cloth surgical gown. **A,** The gown is held by the neck to see the shoulder seams on the inside of the gown. **B,** Close-up of the three seams of one shoulder. **C,** The gown is folded so the outer two seams of one shoulder are touching. **D,** The same fold is done with the other shoulder. **E,** the gown is folded so the seams of both shoulders are touching. **F,** The shoulders are held in one hand while the other hand aligns the armpit seams.

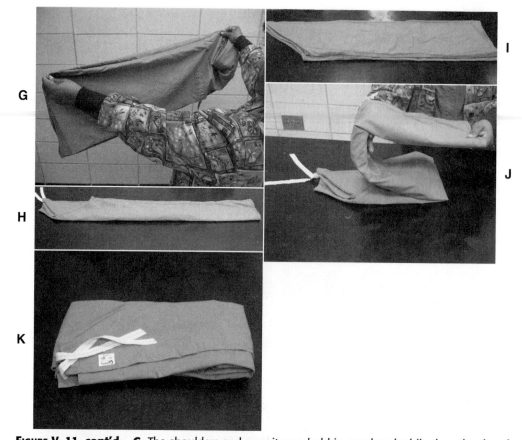

Figure V–11, cont'd **G,** The shoulders and armpits are held in one hand while the other hand aligns the gown hem. **H,** The gown is laid flat on the table. (A tabletop method of folding is to first lay the gown open flat on the countertop with the outside of the gown facing up, sleeves on top. The side edges of the gown are each folded to meet near the middle, and then the gown is folded in half.) Only the inside surfaces of the gown are now exposed. **I,** The gown is folded in half lengthwise. **J,** The gown is folded in accordion fashion. **K,** The gown is laid on the table so the neck ties are uppermost. Proceed to Figure V-13 to wrap the gown.

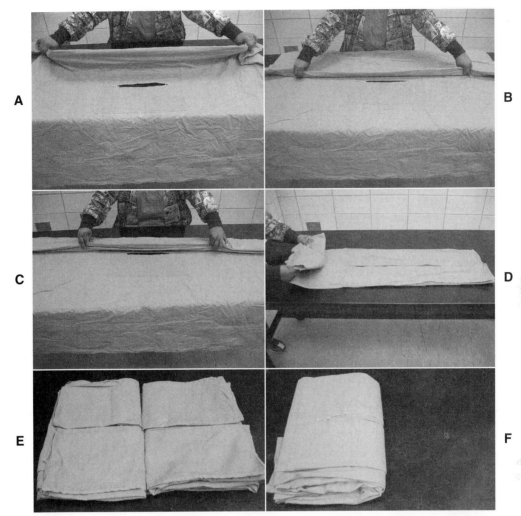

FIGURE V–12 Cloth drapes are folded in accordion fashion so that they are easily unfolded onto the patient. **A** and **B,** A lengthwise fold is created in the drape (approximately 30 cm from the middle), and the folded edge is brought to the fenestration at the middle of the drape. **C,** This is repeated with a second fold, creating an accordion folding. Each secion of folded drape is approximately 15 cm wide. **D,** The opposite side is folded in a similar manner. Then one end of the drape is folded to the center in accordion fashion. **E,** The opposite end is folded in the same manner. **F,** The drape is folded in half (half of the fenestration is visible), and it is ready to be wrapped as in Figure V-13.

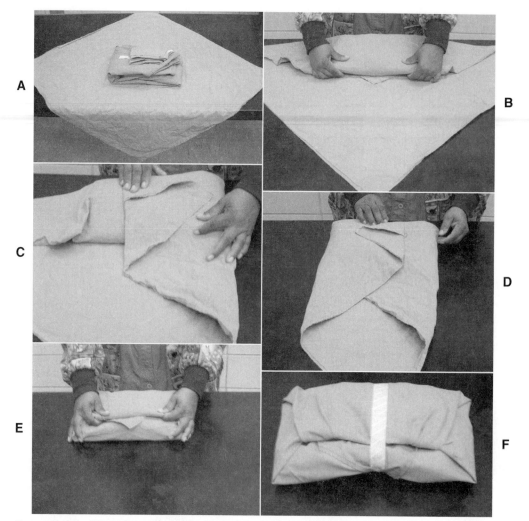

Figure V–13 Wrapping a cloth drape or gown, or an instrument pack. **A,** The gown, along with an accordion-folded hand towel and sterilization indicator, is placed diagonally onto the drapes. **B,** One corner is folded over he entire pack and tucked under it, leaving the tip visible. **C,** An adjacent corner is folded over the end of the pack, and the tip folded back so the drape is flat on top of the pack. **D,** The opposite corner is folded the same way. **E,** The pack is turned around and the final corner is folded over the top of the pack and tucked under the folded drape edges, leaving the tip visible. **F,** The pack is then wrapped in a second layer in the same manner. The pack is secured with autoclave tape and is then labeled with contents, date, and the initials of the individual preparing the pack.

COMPREHENSION QUESTIONS

Directions: Answer the short-answer questions based on the selection. Use the strategies you learned for answering short-answer questions.

1. When folding a surgical gown, the first step is to hold the gown by the _____.

2. In the final step of folding a surgical gown, how is the gown secured? _____

3. How many steps are there in all for folding a surgical gown?_____

4. Why are drapes folded in accordion fashion? _____

_____

5. How wide are the folds for drapes?_____

6. How many steps are there in all for folding drapes? _____

7. What is the first step for the wrapping of a fenestrated drape and gown?

8. What is the following step for the wrapping of a fenestrated drape and gown?

9. How many steps are there in all for the wrapping of a fenestrated drape and gown? _____

10. What labeling is put on the folded drape and gown? _____

WORD PROBLEM

Directions: Use the strategies you learned for solving word problems to answer this question.

Drapes are folded in accordion pleats that are 15 cm wide. If the drape is 120 cm wide, how many folds will be made?

Reading Selection
9

VOCABULARY

Directions: Locate five words that are new to you in this reading. Write the meaning of each of these words in the space provided.

_____

_____

_____

_____

_____

_____

_____

_____

_____

_____

RESPIRATORY DISORDERS

The respiratory system brings oxygen (O_2) into the lungs and removes carbon dioxide (CO_2) from the body. Respiratory disorders interfere with this function and threaten life.

CHRONIC OBSTRUCTIVE PULMONARY DISEASE

Three disorders are grouped under chronic obstructive pulmonary disease (COPD). They are chronic bronchitis, emphysema, and asthma. These disorders interfere with the exchange of O_2 and CO_2 in the lungs. They obstruct airflow.

Chronic Bronchitis. Chronic bronchitis occurs after repeated episodes of bronchitis. Bronchitis means inflammation (*itis*) of the bronchi (*bronch*). Smoking is the major cause. Infection, air pollution, and industrial dusts are other causes.

    Smoker's cough in the morning is often the first symptom. At first the cough is dry. Over time, the person coughs up mucus. Mucus may contain pus. The cough becomes more frequent. The person has difficulty breathing and tires easily. Mucus and inflamed breathing passages obstruct airflow into the lungs. The body cannot get normal amounts of oxygen.

From Sorrentino SA: *Mosby's textbook for nursing assistants*, ed 6, St Louis, 2004, Mosby, pp 690–691.

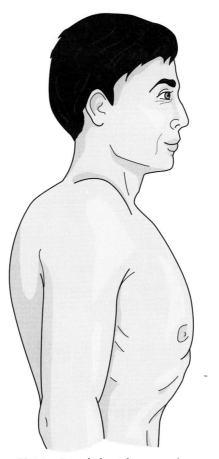

FIGURE V–14   Barrel chest from emphysema.

The person must stop smoking. Oxygen therapy and breathing exercises are often ordered. Respiratory tract infections are prevented. If one occurs, prompt treatment is needed.

Emphysema. In emphysema, the alveoli enlarge. They become less elastic. They do not expand and shrink normally with breathing in and out. As a result, some air is trapped in the alveoli when exhaling. Trapped air is not exhaled. Over time, more alveoli are involved. Therefore more air is trapped. O_2 and CO_2 exchange cannot occur in affected alveoli.

Smoking is the most common cause. The person has shortness of breath and a cough. At first, shortness of breath occurs with exertion. Over time, it occurs at rest. Sputum may contain pus. As more air is trapped in the lungs, the person develops a *barrel chest* (Figure V-14). Breathing is easier when the person sits upright and slightly forward.

The person must stop smoking. Respiratory therapy, breathing exercises, oxygen, and drug therapy are ordered.

Asthma. The airway narrows with asthma. Dyspnea results. Asthma is triggered by allergies and emotional stress. Smoking, respiratory infections, exertion, and cold air are other triggers. Symptoms are mild to severe. Wheezing and coughing are common.

Sudden attacks (*asthma attacks*) can occur. There is shortness of breath, wheezing, coughing, rapid pulse, sweating, and cyanosis. The person gasps for air and is very frightened. Fear makes the attack worse.

Asthma is treated with drugs. Severe attacks may require emergency room treatment. The person and family are taught how to prevent asthma attacks. Repeated attacks can damage the respiratory system.

PNEUMONIA

Pneumonia is an inflammation and infection of lung tissue. Affected tissues fill with fluid. O_2 and CO_2 exchange is affected.

Bacteria, viruses, aspiration, and immobility are causes. The person is very ill. Fever, chills, painful cough, chest pain on breathing, and a rapid pulse occur. Cyanosis may be present. Sputum is thick and green, yellowish, or rust colored. The color depends on the cause.

Drugs are ordered for infection and pain. Fluid intake is increased because of fever. Fluids also thin mucous secretions. Thin secretions are easier to cough up. IV fluids and oxygen may be needed. The person needs plenty of rest. The semi-Fowler's position eases breathing. Standard Precautions are followed. Transmission-Based Precautions are used depending on the cause. Mouth care is important. Frequent linen changes are needed because of fever. *See Focus on Children: Pneumonia. See Focus on Older Persons: Pneumonia.*

WRITING

Directions: Answer the following question based on the reading selection. Remember to use the following writing strategies:

- Organize ideas.
- Write the first draft.
- Revise, edit, and proofread to write the final draft.

Describe the three diseases that affect the organs of respiration.

COMPREHENSION QUESTIONS

Directions: Answer the true and false questions based on the selection. Use the strategies you learned for answering true and false questions.

T   F

____ ____   1. Chronic bronchitis is a type of COPD.

____ ____   2. The airways widen with asthma.

____ ____   3. The causes of asthma are many.

____ ____   4. Chest pain can be a symptom of pneumonia.

____ ____   5. As emphysema progresses, the shortness of breath becomes more severe.

____ ____   6. A patient with asthma has difficulty in breathing.

____ ____   7. Smoking is the most common cause of pneumonia.

____ ____   8. Emphysema is a chronic disease.

____ ____   9. Pneumonia causes a slow pulse.

____ ____   10. The treatment for asthma is medication which closes the air passage-ways.

WORD PROBLEM

Directions: Use the strategies you learned for solving word problems to answer this question.

Timothy Murray had an asthma attack. When he arrived at the hospital at 7:00 AM, the physician noticed that he was wheezing. Timothy said that the wheezing began at 5:30 AM. How long was Timothy experiencing difficulty in breathing?

Reading Selection
10

PREVIEW QUESTION

• What is a pathogen?

VOCABULARY

Directions: Locate five words that are new to you in this reading. Write the meaning of each of these words in the space provided.

_____

_____

_____

_____

_____

_____

_____

_____

_____

_____

THE CHAIN OF INFECTION

The life and growth of **pathogens** (disease-causing organisms) is a *cycle*, or a chain. Break any link in the chain, and you break the infectious process. The chain of infection consists of four parts: (1) virulence, (2) number of microorganisms, (3) susceptible host, and (4) portal of entry (Figure V-15).

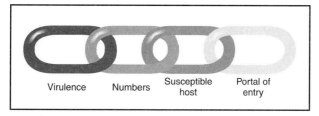

Virulence   Numbers   Susceptible host   Portal of entry

FIGURE V–15   At least one part must be removed to break the chain of infection.

From Bird DL, Robinson DS: *Torres and Ehrlich modern dental assisting*, ed 8, St Louis, 2005, Saunders, pp 278-279.

Virulence

The **virulence** of an organism refers to the degree of *pathogenicity* or strength of that organism in its ability to produce disease. Because the body cannot change the virulence of microorganisms, persons must rely on their body defenses and specific immunizations, such as for hepatitis B virus (HBV). Another defense is to avoid coming in contact with microorganisms by always following the infection-control techniques described in this chapter.

Number of Microorganisms

To cause disease, there must be a high enough number of pathogenic microorganisms present to overwhelm the body's defenses. The number of pathogens may be directly related to the amount of bioburden present. *Bioburden* refers to organic materials such as blood and saliva. The use of the dental dam and high-volume evacuation helps to minimize bioburden on surfaces and thereby reduces the number of microorganisms in the aerosol.

Susceptible Host

A susceptible host is a person who is unable to resist infection by the pathogen. An individual who is in poor health, is chronically fatigued and under extreme stress, or has a weakened immune system is more likely to become infected. Therefore, staying healthy, washing the hands frequently, and keeping immunizations up-to-date will help members of the dental team to resist infection and stay healthy.

Portal of Entry

To cause infection, the pathogens must have a portal of entry, or means of entering the body. The portals of entry for *airborne pathogens* are through the mouth and nose. **Bloodborne pathogens** must have access to the blood supply as a means of entry into the body. This can occur through a break in the skin caused by a needlestick, a cut, or even a human bite. It can also occur through the mucous membranes of the nose and oral cavity.

TYPES OF INFECTIONS

Acute Infection

In an **acute infection,** symptoms are often severe and usually appear soon after the initial infection occurs. Acute infections are of *short duration*. For example, with a viral infection such as the common cold, the body's defense mechanisms usually eliminate the virus within two to three weeks.

Chronic Infection

Chronic infections are those in which the microorganism is present for a *long duration*; some may persist for life. The person may be *asymptomatic* (not showing symptoms of the disease) but may still be a carrier of the disease, as with hepatitis C virus (HCV) or human immunodeficiency virus (HIV) infection.

Latent Infection

A **latent infection** is a persistent infection in which the symptoms "come and go." Cold sores (oral herpes simplex) and genital herpes are latent viral infections.

The virus first enters the body and causes the original lesion. It then lies dormant, away from the surface, in a nerve cell, until certain conditions (such as illness with fever, sunburn, and stress) cause the virus to leave the nerve cell and seek the surface again. Once the virus reaches the surface, it becomes detectable for a short time and causes another outbreak at that site.

Another herpesvirus, *herpes zoster*, causes chickenpox. This virus may lie dormant and later erupt as the painful disease shingles.

Opportunistic Infection

Opportunistic infections are caused by normally nonpathogenic organisms and occur in individuals whose resistance is decreased or compromised. For example, an individual recovering from influenza may develop pneumonia or an ear infection. Opportunistic infections are common in patients with autoimmune disease or diabetes and in elderly persons.

MODES OF DISEASE TRANSMISSION

Before you can prevent disease transmission in the dental office, you must first understand how infectious diseases are spread.

An **infectious disease** is one that is *communicable* or *contagious*. These terms mean that the disease can be transmitted (spread) in some way from one host to another.

Primary Modes of Disease Transmission in Dentistry

Direct contact: Touching or contact with the patient's blood or other body fluids.

Indirect contact: Touching or contact with a contaminated surface or instrument.

Droplet infection: An infection that occurs through mucosal surfaces of the eyes, nose, or mouth.

Parenteral transmission: Needlestick injuries, human bites, cuts, abrasions, or any break in the skin.

WRITING

Directions: Answer the following question based on the reading selection. Remember to use the following writing strategies:

- Organize ideas.
- Write the first draft.
- Revise, edit, and proofread to write the final draft.

Describe six ways in which diseases can be transmitted in the dental office.

COMPREHENSION QUESTIONS

Directions: Answer the matching questions based on the selection. Use the strategies you learned for answering matching questions:

_____ A. Injuries that break the skin.

_____ B. Strength of organism to produce disease.

_____ C. Person unable to resist infection.

_____ D. Touching patient's blood or body fluids.

_____ E. Microorganisms present for a long duration.

_____ F. Symptoms severe, or a short duration.

_____ G. Infection that occurs through mucosal surface of eyes, nose, or mouth.

_____ H. Disease that can be transmitted in some way from one host to another.

_____ I. Cold sores and genital herpes are examples.

_____ J. Touching or contact with a contaminated surface or instrument.

1. Direct contact
2. Communicable disease
3. Indirect contact
4. Latent infection
5. Droplet infection
6. Chronic infection
7. Parenteral transmission
8. Susceptible host
9. Acute infection
10. Virulence

WORD PROBLEM

Directions: Use the strategies you learned for solving word problems to answer this question.

The high-speed handpiece with water spray in a dentist's office produces a mist of bacteria that is equal to having someone sneeze in your face twice per minute. Dr. Michael Peters is exposed to this mist eight hours a day, four days a week. How many sneezes does this mist equal each week?

Reading Selection
11

PREVIEW QUESTION

PREVIEW QUESTION

• Look at figure V-16. What is an intercom?

VOCABULARY

Directions: Locate five words that are new to you in this reading. Write the meaning of each of these words in the space provided.

_____

_____

_____

_____

_____

_____

_____

_____

_____

VOICE MAIL

Many health care facilities, physicians' offices, and homes use voice mail to receive incoming calls. To use voice mail effectively, follow these guidelines.

After listening to the recorded greeting and indicated tone, do the following:

• Speak slowly and distinctly so the person listening to the message can hear and understand what you are communicating.

• If you are leaving a message, include the name of the patient and/or the doctor—give the first and last name, and spell the last name.

• If the message includes a telephone number or laboratory values, speak slowly and repeat the numbers twice, allowing time for the listener to record the information.

• Always leave your name and telephone number, and repeat both twice (at the beginning of the message and at the end of the message) so the listener can call you for clarificaiton if necessary.

From LaFleur Brooks M, Gillingham EA: *Health unit coordinating*, ed 5, St Louis, 2004, Saunders, pp 46-49.

TELEPHONE DIRECTORIES

Many health care facilities publish a directory of extension numbers for telephones in the hospital. They are alphabetized and easy to use. Both department numbers and key personnel are listed. Hospitals using the individual pocket pager also may publish a directory of pocket pager numbers.

The doctors' roster is another directory frequently used by the health unit coordinator. Most health care facilities have computer access to this information, but they also have a hard copy on the nursing units. The information includes the names of the doctors (in alphabetic order) who have admitting or visiting privileges. It lists their medical specialty, their office telephone number, and the answering service telephone number. When placing a telephone call, select the doctor's number with care because there are often several doctors listed with the same name. If two doctors have the same first and last names, refer to their specialty to select the correct telephone number. To practice placing a telephone call, complete the activities at the end of this chapter.

UNIT INTERCOM

The intercom system (Figure V-16) is a device used to communicate between the nurses' station and patients' rooms on a nursing unit. The intercom provides a method of taking patients' requests without going into the room. On admission, the patient should receive directions for the use of the call light and intercom from a member of the nursing staff. The importance of this step is emphasized by the following story: A little boy admitted to a hospital room was not told about the intercom system. When the health unit coordinator noted that the child had his light on, she turned on the intercom and asked if he needed help. He replied, "Yes, wall."

A buzzer and/or light on the intercom alerts you that someone has activated their call system. The room number button lights up on the intercom console to designate the caller's room. By pressing the appropriate button you may converse with the patient. Always identify yourself and your location. For example, you may say, "This is Kimberly at the nurses' station. May I help you?" When there are two or more patients in the room, ask the patient to identify himself or herself.

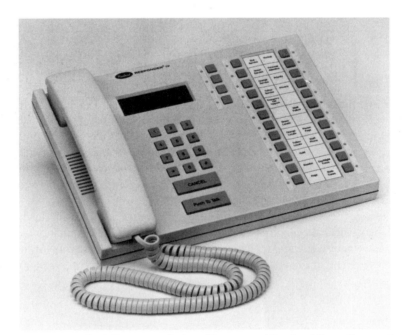

FIGURE V-16 A *Responder* IV intercom device. (Courtesy of Rauland-Borg Corporation.)

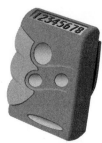

FIGURE V-17   A pocket pager. (Courtesy of Motorola Communications and Electronics, Inc.)

The health unit coordinator also may use the intercom to locate nursing personnel. To page personnel on the intercom, depress the button that allows for the message to be heard in each of the rooms. A simple message, such as "Susan, please call the nurses' station," is all that is needed.

The health unit coordinator should be selective in the information communicated over the intercom because some types of messages may prove embarrassing to the patient. For example, do not use the intercom to ask a patient if he or she has had a bowel movement. Try to keep the message as brief as possible, and do not communicate any confidential patient information to a nurse over the intercom because other patients may hear the message.

POCKET PAGER

The pocket pager (Figure V-17) is a small, electronic device that is activated by dialing a series of numbers on a telephone to deliver a message to the carrier of the pager. The pocket pager may be digital or voice. When using a voice pager, dial the pager number and state the message. Always say the message including name and extension number twice. A digital pager is similar in appearance to a voice pager. To contact a person by digital pager, dial the pager number from a touch-tone phone. Listen for a ring followed by a series of beeps. Dial your telephone number followed by the pound sign (#). You will hear a series of fast beeps, which indicates a completed page. The number appears on the pager display. The receiver then calls you back for the message. Allow at least 5 minutes before paging a second time, unless it is a stat (emergency) situation.

Some nursing units use a number code entered at the end of the call back number—the number 1 indicating "stat," number 2 indicating "as soon as possible," and number 3 indicating "at your convenience." Residents, ancillary personnel, and your instructor carry pocket pagers.

VOICE PAGING SYSTEM

The voice paging system is a communication system in which the hospital switchboard operator, upon request, pages someone on a speaker that is heard in every area of the hospital. To locate a doctor with this system, dial the hospital switchboard operator, indicate the name of the doctor who is needed, and give the telephone extension number of the unit you are on. The operator announces the name of the doctor needed and the extension number to call.

The operator also uses the voice paging system to locate a doctor for calls from outside the hospital. The health unit coordinator frequently is asked by doctors to listen for their page, especially when they are in a patient's room. When a page for a doctor is announced, the health unit coordinator may contact the operator for the message and deliver it to the doctor.

COPY AND SHREDDER MACHINES

Many nursing units have a copy machine available for making copies of written or typed materials. Photocopying of patient records is discussed in Chapter 6. The fax machine also can be used to make a minimal amount of copies.

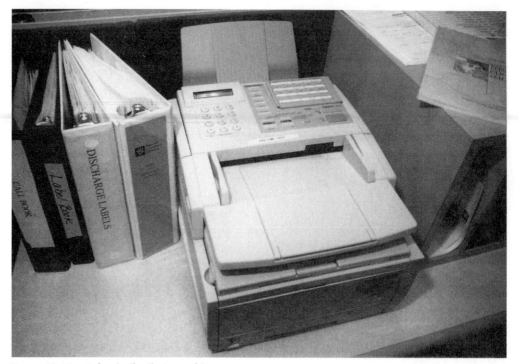

FIGURE V-18 A facsimile (fax) machine.

Patient forms containing confidential information cannot be thrown in the wastebasket. Shredder machines or boxes for materials to be picked up and taken to be shredded are placed on nursing units. Chart forms that have labels with patient name, patient account number, and health record identification number that do not have documentation on them must be shredded.

FAX MACHINE

A fax machine is a telecommunication device that transmits copies of written material over a telephone wire from one site to another (Figure V-18). Reports and other documents are faxed to and from health care institutions and doctors' offices. Most hospitals, to be cost effective, have eliminated the three part (NCR, or no carbon required) physician order sheets in favor of faxing the orders to the pharmacy. When faxing the pharmacy copy, the health unit coordinator can use the fax machine to make a copy of the orders to give to the appropriate nurse. Fax machines have a redial option, allowing a document to be sent to the location last programmed into the machine. Many health care workers in the nurses' station use the fax machine. Therefore, it is important not to use the redial option that may send a document to the wrong location. Patient information is extremely confidential and if sent to the wrong location could result in an employee being disciplined or terminated. The fax machine is not for personal use, such as sending jokes to coworkers, entries in contests, or the like.

PNEUMATIC TUBE

The pneumatic tube is a system in which air pressure transports tubes carrying supplies, requisitions, or messages from one hospital unit or department to another. These items are placed in a special carrying tube, which then is inserted into the pneumatic tube system; a keypad is used to enter the location to where the message is to be sent. Medications that do not break or spill are transported in this manner. Do *not* place specimens obtained by a painful procedure in the pneumatic tube. When a tube carrying supplies or other items arrives at the nursing unit, it is the health unit coordinator's responsibility to remove the tube from the pneumatic tube system as soon as possible and disperse the items accordingly. You will be instructed in the operation of your hospital's pneumatic tube system during your hospital orientation.

Some health care facilities have a telelift system that is operated in much the same way and for the same purposes as the tube system. It consists of a small boxcar that is carried on a conveyor belt to designated locations. A keypad is used to program the car to go to a specific unit of a department.

WRITING

Directions: Answer the following question based on the reading selection. Remember to use the following writing strategies:

- Organize ideas.
- Write the first draft.
- Revise, edit, and proofread to write the final draft.

Which features of editing text with a word processing program would be particularly helpful to you? Explain why.

COMPREHENSION QUESTIONS

Directions: Answer the short-answer questions based on the selection. Use the strategies you learned for answering short-answer questions.

1. Do not use the _____ function when using a fax machine.

2. Patient forms containing _____ information cannot be thrown in the wastebasket.

3. A system that uses air pressure to transport supplies, requisitions, or messages is a _____ tube.

4. A telecommunications device that transmits copies of written material over a telephone line is a _____.

5. A buzzer and/or light can alert you that someone has activated their call system on a _____.

6. When using _____, you should speak slowly and distinctly.

7. When two doctors have the same name, refer to their _____ to select the correct phone number.

8. You should always leave your name and telephone number when leaving a voice mail message and repeat them both_____.

9. A _____ is used to page an individual on a speaker that is heard in every area of the hospital.

10. Confidential patient information must be _____.

WORD PROBLEM

Directions: Use the strategies you learned for solving word problems to answer this question.

Julie Sands has been editing text with the word processor for 2 hours. It used to take her half of her 8-hour working day to edit the same amount of text with her typewriter. How many hours longer did editing with a typewriter take than editing with a word processor?

Reading Selection
12

VOCABULARY

Directions: Locate five words that are new to you in this reading. Write the meaning of each of these words in the space provided.

_____

_____

_____

_____

_____

_____

_____

_____

_____

_____

THE SURGERY CONSENT

The person's consent is needed before surgery is done. An *operative permit* or *surgical consent* is signed when the person understands the information given by the doctor. The person's spouse or nearest relative may be required to sign the consent. A parent or legal guardian signs for a minor child. The legal guardian signs for a person who is mentally incompetent.

The doctor is responsible for securing written consent. Often this is delegated to an RN. *You do not obtain the person's written consent for surgery.*

THE PREOPERATIVE CHECKLIST

A preoperative checklist is placed on the front of the person's chart. When the list is complete, the person is ready for surgery. The nurse may ask you to do some things on the list. Promptly report when you complete each task. Also report any observations. Except for the bed rails, the entire checklist is completed before preoperative drugs are given.

From Sorrentino SA: *Mosby's textbook for nursing assistants*, ed 6, St Louis, 2004, Mosby, p 570.

Marking the surgical site. Many agencies mark the surgical site. This is to prevent surgery on the wrong body part. Sometimes the patient marks the body part. This is done as part of the preoperative checklist. It is done before preoperative drugs are given.

PREOPERATIVE MEDICATION

About 45 minutes to 1 hour before surgery, the preoperative drugs are given. They are given to:

- Help the person relax and feel drowsy
- Reduce respiratory secretions to prevent aspiration
- Prevent nausea and vomiting

The person feels sleepy and lightheaded. Thirst and dry mouth also occur. Falls and accidents are prevented after the drugs are given. Bed rails are raised. The person is not allowed out of bed. Therefore the person voids before the drugs are given. After they are given, the bedpan or urinal is used for voiding.

After the drugs are given, move furniture to make room for the stretcher. Also clean off the overbed table and the bedside stand. This prevents damage to equipment and valuables. Raise the bed to its highest level to transfer the patient from the bed to a stretcher.

TRANSPORT TO THE OPERATING ROOM

An OR staff member brings a stretcher to the room. The patient is transferred to the stretcher and covered with a bath blanket. The blanket provides warmth and prevents exposure. Falls are prevented. Safety straps are secured and the side rails raised. A pillow is placed under the person's head for comfort.

Identification checks are made. Then the person's chart is given to the OR staff member. The person is transported to the OR. The family may be allowed to go as far as the OR entrance. See *Focus on Children: Transport to the Operating Room.*

ANESTHESIA

Anesthesia is the loss of feeling or sensation produced by a drug. These types of anesthesia are common:

- **General anesthesia** is the loss of consciousness and all feeling or sensation. A drug is given IV, or a gas is inhaled.
- **Regional anesthesia** is the loss of feeling or sensation in a large area of the body. The person is awake. A drug is injected into a body part.
- **Local anesthesia** is the loss of feeling or sensation in a small area. A drug is injected at the site.
- Anesthetics are given by specially educated doctors and nurses. An *anesthesiologist* is a doctor who specializes in giving anesthetics. An *anesthetist* is an RN with advanced study giving anesthetics.

WRITING

Directions: Answer the following question based on the reading selection. Remember to use the following writing strategies:

- Organize ideas.
- Write the first draft.
- Revise, edit, and proofread to write the final draft.

What are the differences in the three types of anesthesia?

COMPREHENSION QUESTIONS

Directions: Answer the multiple-choice questions based on the selection. Use the strategies you learned for answering multiple-choice questions.

1. An anesthesiologist is a
   a. registered nurse
   b. a physician
   c. a medication
   d. an illness

2. General anesthesia is a
   a. body organ
   b. spinal tap
   c. loss of consciousness
   d. deep wound

3. An anesthetist is a/n _____ with advanced study giving anesthetics
   a. RN
   b. doctor
   c. a nursing assistant
   d. a medical assistant

4. Preoperative medication is given _____ surgery
   a. during
   b. before
   c. after
   d. none of the above

5. The anesthesia which is injected directly into the surgical area is
   a. local
   b. regional
   c. general
   d. ineffective

6. A consent for a minor child is signed
   a. by the child
   b. by the physician
   c. by a parent or guardian
   d. by the nursing assistant

7. Loss of feeling in a large area of the body is caused by
   a. a relaxing medication
   b. general anesthesia
   c. local anesthesia
   d. regional anesthesia

8. A loss of sensation is called
   a. anesthesia
   b. anesthesiologist
   c. anesthetist
   d. sutures

9. Surgical sites are marked _____ preoperative drugs are given
   a. after
   b. at the same time
   c. before
   d. unless

10. When regional anesthesia is administered
    a. the drug is inhaled
    b. the patient loses consciousness
    c. the patient is awake
    d. the patient can move only the upper extremities

WORD PROBLEM

Directions: Use the strategies you learned for solving word problems to answer this question.

The anesthetist planned to administer anesthesia to the patient 70 minutes before surgery. The surgery was scheduled for 3:00 PM. What time was the anesthesia administered?

Reading Selection
13

PREVIEW QUESTION

• What specific injuries can be caused by electrical burns?

VOCABULARY

Directions: Locate five words that are new to you in this reading. Write the meaning of each of these words in the space provided.

_____

_____

_____

_____

_____

_____

_____

_____

_____

_____

ELECTRICAL BURNS

In the United States, about 1,000 people die each year from electrical injuries. At high risk are industrial workers and children. Electrical incidents occur as a result of downed power lines, the malfunctioning of home appliances, children chewing through electrical lines, accidental contact with television antennae by unskilled individuals, and contact with high-tension power lines.

When electricity traverses the body, it is converted to heat that burns the tissues in its path. High-voltage arcs generate intense amounts of heat and can burn a person nearby. Death can result from the passage of current through vital organs, which causes respiratory or cardiac arrest.

From Henry MC, Stapleton ER: *EMT prehospital care*, ed 3, St Louis, 2004, Mosby/JEMS, pp 597-599.

EMT's must take precautions to protect themselves and the patient from further injury. Knowing some basic properties of electricity may help guide you to take correct actions.

Electricity is the movement of electrons from a point of higher concentration to a point of lower concentration. Electricity is often described in terms of three variables:

- Amperage is the number or volume of electrons flowing.
- Voltage is the force with which movement occurs.
- Resistance is the degree of hindrance to electron flow.

These three concepts are interrelated by the formula

$$A \text{ (amperage)} = \frac{V \text{ (voltage)}}{R \text{ (resistance)}}$$

Current can be direct or unidirectional in flow or it can alternate or switch the direction of electron flow at a given number of cycles per second (hertz). Flow from a battery is an example of direct current; household electrical flow is usually a form of alternating current.

Generally, exposure to low voltage is less serious than to high voltage. However, fatalities have occurred with voltage as low as 45 to 60 Hz. Household current is capable of causing a sustained muscular contraction preventing release of the electrified object by the patient. Amperage, which is not usually known, also does more damage as the number of milliamperes increases. Symptoms can range from tingling to sustained muscular contraction to fatal organ damage. If current passes through the brain, it may cause respiratory arrest. If it passes through the heart, it may cause cardiac arrest.

Resistance is defined as a measure of the hindrance to electron flow through a given material. Materials vary tremendously in their resistance. For example, copper wires offer relatively low resistance and conduct electricity readily; they serve as good conductors. Rubber has a very high resistance to electrical flow; it serves as an insulator. Good conductors offer low resistance. Poor conductors offer high resistance. Lightning rods, for instance, are made of metal, which is a good conductor, and are used to direct electricity from the roof of a house along insulated wires to the ground. Because electricity seeks to flow along the path of least resistance from a higher to a lower potential, lightning rods prevent electricity from traveling through a highly resistant wooden roof, which would generate heat and fire. Instead, the electricity is directed to the earth, which can absorb the current.

Vehicles are insulated from the ground by their rubber tires. Thus a downed power line in contact with a vehicle may leave the occupants unharmed as long as they avoid direct contact with the ground. However, if they step out of the car while holding onto the door, they will be part of the circuit consisting of the wire, the vehicle, their bodies, and the ground, and they will sustain electrical injury.

When electrical current passes through the body as part of its circuit (usually to the ground), it follows an internal path of least resistance. Skin and bone offer high resistance to electrical current, muscle offers less, and the vessels and nerves offer the least resistance to electrical flow. Therefore, current passing from arm to arm tends to pass along the vessels and nerves in the arms and thorax. Even high current can enter and exit at relatively small surface areas; you therefore cannot gauge the extent of internal injury from the external appearance.

Wet skin, offering less resistance, is more easily penetrated by electricity than dry skin. Even household current that penetrates wet skin can cause cardiac arrest.

Burns to the soft tissues, because of the heat generated from electric current, can extend from superficial to full-thickness burns. Full-thickness burns can vary from those that look gray-white to those that appear charred. Thermal burns can also be caused by the intense heat generated by electrical arcs that are nearby but not in direct contact with the body. In general, the longer the duration of contact, the greater the severity of the burn. Electrical burns tend to be more extensive than they appear, as judged from their external marks.

The most immediate life-threatening effects of electrical injuries are respiratory and cardiac arrest. Early resuscitation can improve patient outcome. For example, respiratory arrest after a lightning injury can be prolonged, but patients who have received early respiratory support have recovered. Associated falls may cause fractures and other injuries. Lightning injuries also burn the skin and soft tissue.

ASSESSMENT AND TREATMENT

The first priority is to assess whether hazards continue to exist. Are there fallen wires? Any downed wire should be considered as charged until the appropriate authorities, such as power company personnel, confirm that the power is off. Rescuers should not attempt to secure power lines with a stick or rope or other nonconductive material because the risk of injury to the rescuer is high.

When encountering victims trapped in a vehicle in contact with a downed wire, have them remain in the vehicle. Do not touch the vehicle or patient yourself because that will place you in a circuit from the vehicle to the ground. If there is a fire in the vehicle, patients should jump out or throw small children to rescue personnel (making sure there is never a circuit from the car to the ground).

After ensuring rescuer safety, assess and manage any life-threatening conditions with appropriate concern for the cervical spine if falls or violent contractions have occurred. Look closely for any fractures and splint appropriately. When assessing the skin, look for both entrance and exit wounds. Cover the wounds with sterile dressings and transport the patient to the hospital.

WRITING

Directions: Answer the following question based on the reading selection. Remember to use the following writing strategies:

- Organize ideas.
- Write the first draft.
- Revise, edit, and proofread to write the final draft.

What should the EMT know about electricity to protect the burn victim from further injury?

COMPREHENSION QUESTIONS

Directions: Answer the true and false questions based on the selection. Use the strategies you learned for answering true and false questions.

T F

1. Wet skin is more easily penetrated by electricity than dry skin.
2. In the United States, 10,000 people die each year from electrical injuries.
3. Death can result from the passage of current through vital organs.
4. A=V/R
5. Exposure to low voltage is more serious than exposure to high voltage.
6. Burns to the soft tissue extend from superficial to full thickness burns.

_____ _____ 7. Amperage is the number or volumes of electrons flowing.
_____ _____ 8. Downed wire should be considered as charged.
_____ _____ 9. Cars are insulated from the ground by their rubber tires.
_____ _____ 10. If a current passes through the heart, it will always cause cardiac arrest.

WORD PROBLEM

Directions: Use the strategies you learned for solving word problems to answer this question.

Fatalities can occur with voltage as low as 45 to 60 cycles per second. If the voltage is 90 to 120 cycles per second, how much greater is the risk?

Reading Selection
14

PREVIEW QUESTION
- What is another name for amyotrophic lateral sclerosis?

VOCABULARY

Directions: Locate five words that are new to you in this reading. Write the meaning of each of these words in the space provided.

_____

_____

_____

_____

_____

_____

_____

_____

_____

DEGENERATIVE, MOVEMENT, AND SEIZURE DISORDERS
Alzheimer Disease (AD)

Brain disorder marked by gradual deterioration of mental capacity (dementia) beginning in middle age.

An early sign is loss of memory for recent events, persons, and places, followed by impairment of judgment, comprehension, and intellect. Anxiety, depression, and emotional disturbances occur as well. On autopsy there is atrophy of the cerebral cortex and widening of the cerebral sulci, especially in the frontal and temporal regions (Figure V-19). Microscopic examination shows **senile plaques** resulting from degeneration of neurons and **neurofibrillary tangles** (bundles of fibrils in the cytoplasm of a neuron) in the cerebral cortex. Deposits of **amyloid** (a protein) occur in neurofibrillary tangles, senile plaques and in blood vessels. The cause of AD remains unknown, although genetic factors may play a role. A mutation on chromosome 14 has been linked to familial cases. There is as yet no effective treatment.

From Chabner DE: *The language of medicine*, ed 7, St Louis, 2004, Saunders, pp 354-356.

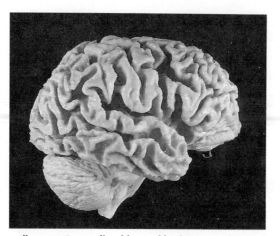

FIGURE V-19 Alzheimer disease. Generalized loss of brain parenchyma (neuronal tissue) results in the narrowing of the cerebral cortical gyri and the widening of the sulci.

Amyotrophic Lateral Sclerosis (ALS)

Degenerative disease of motor neurons in the spinal cord and brainstem; motor neuron disease.

ALS presents in adulthood and affects men more often than women. Symptoms are weakness and atrophy of muscles in the hands, forearms, and legs, followed by difficulty in swallowing, talking, and dyspnea as the respiratory muscles become affected. Etiology (cause) and cure for ALS are both unknown.

A famous baseball player, Lou Gehrig, became a victim of this disease in the mid 1900s and thus the condition was known as Lou Gehrig disease.

Epilepsy

Chronic brain disorder characterized by recurrent seizure activity.

A seizure is an abnormal, sudden excessive discharge of electrical activity within the brain. Seizures are often symptom of underlying brain pathological conditions, such as brain tumors, meningitis, vascular disease, or scar tissue from a head injury. **Tonic-clonic seizures (ictal events)** are characterized by a sudden loss of consciousness, falling down, and then tonic contractions (stiffening of muscles) followed by clonic contractions (twitching and jerking movements of the limbs). These convulsions are often preceded by an **aura**, which is a peculiar sensation appearing before more definite symptoms. Dizziness, numbness, or visual disturbances are examples of an aura. **Absence seizures (petit mal seizures)** are a minor form of seizure consisting of momentary clouding of consciousness and loss of contact with the environment. Drug therapy (anticonvulsants) is used for control of epileptic seizures.

After seizures, there may be neurologic symptoms such as weakness; called **postictal events**. Epilepsy comes from the Greek *epilepsis*, meaning "a laying hold of." The Greeks thought a victim of a seizure was laid hold of by some mysterious force.

Huntington Disease

Hereditary nervous disorder caused by degenerative changes in the cerebrum and involving bizarre, abrupt, involuntary, dance-like movements.

This condition begins in adulthood (between the ages of 30 and 45) and results in personality changes with choreic (meaning dance) movements (uncontrollable, irregular, jerking movements of the arms, legs, and face).

The genetic defect in patients with Huntington disease is located on chromosome 4. Patients can be tested for the gene; however, no cure exists and management is symptomatic.

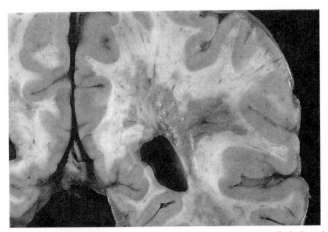

FIGURE V-20   Multiple sclerosis (MS). The typical MS plaque is a well-defined, grey-pink lesion that can occur anywhere in the brain or spinal cord. Common sites are the white matter around the ventricles of the brain, the optic nerves, and the white matter of the spinal cord. (From Kumar V, Cotran RS, Robbins SL: Basic Pathology, ed 7, Philadelphia, Saunders, 2003, pp. 843 and 838.)

Multiple Sclerosis (MS)

Destruction of the myelin sheath on neurons in the CNS and its replacement by plaques of sclerotic (hard) tissue (Figure V-20).

One of the leading causes of neurological disability in persons 20 to 40 years of age, MS is a chronic disease often marked by long periods of stability (remission) and worsening (relapse). **Demyelination** (loss of myelin insulation) prevents the conduction of nerve impulses through the axon and causes paresthesias, muscle weakness, unsteady **gait** (manner of walking), and paralysis. There may be visual (blurred and double vision) and speech disturbances as well. Etiology is unknown, but it is likely to be an autoimmune or viral disease in which lymphoctyes react against myelin. Immunosuppressive agents (interferon, steroids, or chemotherapy) are often given with benefit.

Myasthenia Gravis

Neuromuscular disorder characterized by weakness (asthenia) of voluntary muscles (attached to bones).

Myasthenia gravis means "grave muscle weakness" and is a chronic autoimmune disorder. Antibodies block the ability of acetylcholine (neurotransmitter) to transmit the nervous impulse from nerve to muscle cell. Normal muscle contraction fails to occur. Onset of symptoms is usually gradual with ptosis of the upper eyelid, double vision (diplopia), and facial weakness. Therapy to reverse symptoms includes anticholinesterase drugs, which inhibit the enzyme that breaks down acetylcholine. Corticosteroids (prednisone) and immunosuppressive drugs (azathioprine, methotrexate, and cyclophosphamide) are also used in treatment. **Thymectomy** (removal of the thymus gland, the source of antibodies against nerve impulse transmission) is an alternative method of treatment and is beneficial to many patients.

Palsy

Paralysis (partial or complete loss of motor function).

Cerebral palsy is partial paralysis and lack of muscular coordination caused by loss of oxygen (hypoxia) or blood flow to the cerebrum during gestation or in the perinatal period. **Bell palsy** is paralysis on one side of the face. Etiology is likely infection with a virus, and therapy is directed against the virus (antivirals) and nerve swelling.

Parkinson Disease (Parkinsonism)

Degeneration of nerves in the basal ganglia, occurring in later life and leading to tremors, weakness of muscles, and slowness of movement.

This slowly progressive condition is caused by a deficiency of dopamine (neurotransmitter) made by cells in the basal ganglia. Motor disturbances include stooped posture, shuffling gait, muscle stiffness (rigidity), and often a tremor of the hands.

Drugs such as levodopa plus carbidopa (Sinemet) to increase dopamine levels in the brain are **palliative** (relieving symptoms but not curative) measures. Implantation of fetal brain tissue containing dopamine-producing cells is an experimental treatment but has produced uncertain results.

Tourette Syndrome

Involuntary, spasmodic, twitching movements; uncontrollable vocal sounds; and inappropriate words.

These involuntary movements, usually beginning with twitching of the eyelid and muscles of the face with verbal outbursts, are called **tics**. Although the cause of Tourette syndrome is not known, it is associated with either an excess of dopamine or a hypersensitivity to dopamine. Psychological problems do not cause Tourette syndrome, but physicians have had some success in treating it with the antipsychotic drug haloperidol (Haldol), antidepressants, and mood stablizers.

WRITING

Directions: Answer the following questions based on the reading selection. Remember to use the following writing strategies:

- Organize ideas.
- Write the first draft.
- Revise, edit, and proofread to write the final draft.

What are the signs of Alzheimer's disease? How do these signs differ from Parkinson's disease?

COMPREHENSION QUESTIONS

Directions: Answer the short-answer questions based on the selection. Use the strategies you learned for answering short-answer questions.

1. Dementia is the gradual _____ of mental capacity.
2. Lou Gehrig was a famous _____.
3. _____ is marked by abnormal, sudden excessive discharge of electrical activity within the brain.
4. Bell's palsy is paralysis on _____.
5. Neurologic symptoms occurring after a seizure are _____ events.
6. The genetic defect in patients with Huntington's disease is located on chromosome _____.
7. The removal of the thymus gland is called a _____.
8. Parkinson's disease is a _____ of nerves in the brain.
9. _____ is partial or complete loss of motor function.
10. Drugs that relieve but do not cure are called _____.

WORD PROBLEM

Directions: Use the strategies you learned for solving word problems to answer this question.

A class training to become nursing assistants was taught the signs of MS. Two-thirds of the students were able to recognize those patients who had this disease. If there are 30 students, how many still have to learn to recognize the signs of MS?

Reading Selection
15

PREVIEW QUESTION
- What does COPD stand for?

VOCABULARY

Directions: Locate five words that are new to you in this reading. Write the meaning of each of these words in the space provided.

_____

_____

_____

_____

_____

_____

_____

_____

_____

PHARMACOLOGICAL MANAGEMENT OF CHRONIC OBSTRUCTIVE PULMONARY DISEASE

Definition of Chronic Obstructive Pulmonary Disease

Chronic obstructive pulmonary disease (COPD) is a disease state characterized by airflow limitation that is not fully reversible. The airflow limitation is usually both progressive and associated with an abnormal inflammatory response of the lungs to noxious particles or gases.

From Rau JL: *Respiratory care pharmacology*, ed 6, St Louis, 2002, Mosby, pp 472-473.

TABLE 15-1   Classification of Chronic Obstructive Pulmonary Disease by Severity

Stage	Characteristics
0: At risk	Normal spirometry; chronic symptoms (cough, sputum production)
I: Mild COPD	FEV1*/FVC <70% FEV1 ≥80% predicted With or without chronic symptoms (cough, sputum production)

II: Moderate COPD	FEV1/FVC <70%
	    IIA: 50% £FEV1 <80% predicted
	    IIB: 30% £FEV1 <50% predicted
	With or without chronic symptoms (cough, sputum production, dyspnea)

III: Severe COPD	FEV1/FVC <70% FEV1 <30% predicted or FEV1 <50% predicted plus respiratory failure† or clinical signs of right heart failure

From Global Initiative for Chronic Obstructive Lung Disease (GOLD), Workshop Report: *Global strategy for the diagnosis, management, and prevention of COPD,* Bethesda, Md, 2000, National Heart, Lung, and Blood Institute and the World Health Organization.
COPD, Chronic obstructive pulmonary disease; FEV_1, forced expiratory volume in 1 second; FVC, forced vital capacity.
*All FEV_1 values in the GOLD Workshop Report refer to postbronchodilator FEV_1.
†Respiratory failure: Pao_2 less than 8.0 kPa (60 mm Hg) with or without $Paco_2$ greater than 6.7 kPa (50 mm Hg) while breathing air at sea level.

Goals of Long-Term Management of Chronic Obstructive Pulmonary Disease

- Prevent disease progression
- Relieve symptoms (dyspnea, cough, fatigue)
- Improve exercise tolerance
- Improve health status
- Prevent and treat complications
- Prevent and treat exacerbations
- Reduce mortality

GENERAL MANAGEMENT OF STABLE CHRONIC OBSTRUCTIVE PULMONARY DISEASE

The overall approach to management in stable COPD is a stepwise increase in treatment depending on the severity of the disease.

- Health education, including smoking cessation
- Pharmacological management
- Exercise training programs to improve exercise tolerance and reduce symptoms of dyspnea and fatigue
- Long-term oxygen (> 15 hours per day) to patients with chronic respiratory failure

Pharmacological Treatment of Stable Chronic Obstructive Pulmonary Disease

None of the existing medications for COPD has been shown to modify the long-term decline in lung function. Pharmacological therapy is used to prevent and control symptoms, reduce the frequency and severity of exacerbations, and improve health status and exercise tolerance. The following table summarizes the GOLD guidelines for treatment at each stage of COPD. *The complete GOLD Guidelines should be consulted for more detail in drug management of COPD.*

Therapy at Each Stage of Chronic Obstructive Pulmonary Disease

Patients must be taught how and when to use their treatments, and treatments being prescribed for other conditions should be reviewed. β-Blocking agents (including eye drop formulations) should be avoided.

TABLE 15-2 Therapy at Each Stage of Chronic Obstructive Pulmonary Disease

Stage	Characteristic	Recommended Treatment
All		Avoidance of risk factor(s) Influenza vaccination
0: At risk	Chronic symptoms (cough, sputum) Exposure to risk factors Normal spirometry	
I: Mild COPD	FEV_1/FVC <70% FEV_1 ≥80% predicted with or without symptoms	Short-acting bronchodilator when needed
II: Moderate COPD	FEV_1/FVC < 70% IIA: 50% ≤FEV_1 <80% predicted with or without symptoms	Regular treatment with one or more bronchodilators Rehabilitation Inhaled glucocorticoids if significant symptoms and lung function response*
	IIB: 30% ≤FEV_1 <50% predicted with or without symptoms	Regular treatment with one or more bronchodilators Rehabilitation Inhaled glucocorticoids if significant symptoms and lung function response* or if repeated exacerbations
III: Severe COPD	FEV_1/FVC < 70% FEV_1 < 30% predicted or respiratory failure† or clinical signs of right heart failure	Regular treatment with one or more bronchodilators Inhaled glucocorticoids if significant symptoms and lung function response* or if repeated exacerbations Treatment of complications Rehabilitation Long-term oxygen therapy if respiratory failure Consider surgical treatments

COPD, Chronic obstruction pulmonary disease; *FEV_1*, forced expiratory volume in 1 second; *FVC_1*, forced vital capacity.
*Criteria for response: trial of inhaled glucocorticosteroids for 6 weeks to 3 months, with an increaase in FEV_1 of 200 ml and 15% of the postbronchodilator response baseline.
†Respiratory failure: Pao_2 less than 8.0 kPa (60 mm Hg) with or without $Paco_2$ greater than kPa (50 mm Hg) while breathing air at sea level.

The GOLD Guidelines provide the following comments on each class of drug therapy in stable COPD.

Bronchodilators

- Bronchodilator medications are central to symptom management in COPD.
- Inhaled therapy is preferred (theophylline is effective in COPD, but because of potential toxicity, inhaled bronchodilators are preferred when available.)

- The choice between β_2-agonist, anticholinergic, theophylline, or combination therapy depends on availability and individual reponse in terms of symptom relief and side effects.
- Bronchodilators are prescribed on an as needed or a regular basis to prevent or reduce symptoms.
- Long-acting inhaled bronchodilators are more convenient.
- Combining bronchodilators may improve efficacy and decrease the risk of side effects compared with increasing the dose of a single bronchodilator.

Glucocorticoids

- Regular treatment with inhaled glucocorticosteroids is only appropriate for symptomatic COPD patients with a documented spirometric response to inhaled glucocorticosteroids, or in those with an FEV_1 less than 50% of predicted (Stage IIB: Moderate COPD and Stage III: Severe COPD) and repeated exacerbations requiring treatment with antibiotics or oral glucocorticosteroids.
- Long-term treatment with oral glucocorticosteroids is not recommended in management of stable COPD.

Other Pharmacological Treatments

- **Vaccines:** Influenza vaccines are recommended; pneumococcal vaccine lacks sufficient data to support general use in COPD.
- **α_1-Antitrypsin augmentation therapy:** This therapy is recommended in young patients with severe hereditary α_1-antitrypsin deficiency and established emphysema; not recommended for COPD unrelated to α_1-antitrypsin deficiency.
- **Antibiotics:** Use of antibiotics other than to treat infectious exacerbations and other bacterial infections is not recommended.
- **Mucolytic (mucokinetic and mucoregulator) agents:** A few patients with viscous sputum may benefit from mucolytics, although overall benefits seem to be small; not recommended for widespread use. This group includes agents such as ambroxol, erdosteine, carbocysteine, iodinated glycerol.
- **Antioxidant agents:** Antioxidants, particularly *N*-acetylcysteine, have been shown to reduce the frequency of exacerbations and may be useful in patients with recurrent exacerbations. Additional studies needed for recommending in routine treatment.
- **Antitussives:** Regular use of antitussives is contraindicated in stable COPD.
- **Vasodilators:** In stable COPD, inhaled nitric oxide can worsen gas exchange and is contraindicated.
- **Respiratory stimulants:** Use of either intravenous doxapram or almitrine bismesylate is not recommended in stable COPD.
- **Narcotics:** These agents are contraindicated in COPD because of their respiratory depressant effects.
- **Others:** Nedocromil, leukotriene modifiers, or alternative healing methods (e.g., herbal medicine, acupuncture, homeopathy) have not been adequately tested in COPD patients and cannot be recommended at this time.

MANAGEMENT OF EXACERBATIONS

The complete GOLD Guidelines should be consulted for more detail in management of COPD exacerbations.

Home Management

The GOLD Guidelines note that when to treat an exacerbation at home and when to hospitalize a patient is a major outstanding issue.

Bronchodilator Therapy

- Increase dose and frequency of existing bronchodilator therapy.
- If not already used, add an anticholinergic agent until symptoms improve.
- High-dose nebulized therapy can be given on an as-needed basis for several days.

Glucocorticosteroids

- Consider if patient's baseline FEV_1 is less than 50% predicted. A dose of prednisolone 40 mg per day for 10 days is recommended.

Antibiotics

Only effective when patients with worsening dyspnea and cough have increased sputum volume and purulence. Choice of agents should reflect local patterns of antibiotic sensitivity among *S. pneumoniae*, *H. influenzae*, and *M. catarrhalis*.

Hospital Management

- Assess severity of symptoms, blood gases, chest x-ray.
  - If life-threatening (development of respiratory acidosis, significant comorbidities, and the need for ventilatory support), admit directly to ICU.
- Adminsiter controlled oxygen therapy; repeat arterial blood gas measurement after 30 minutes.
- Bronchodilators:
  - Increase doses or frequency.
  - Combine β_2-agonists and anticholinergics.
  - Use spacers or air-driven nebulizers.
  - Consider adding intravenous methylxanthine, if needed.
- Add oral or intravenous glucocorticosteroids.
- Consider antibiotics when signs of bacterial infection (worsening dyspnea, cough, increased sputum volume and purulence); oral or occasionally intravenous.
- Consider noninvasive mechanical ventilation.
- At all times:
  - Monitor fluid balance and nutrition.
  - Consider subcutaneous heparin.
  - Identify and treat associated conditions (e.g., heart failure, arrhythmias).
  - Closely monitor condition of the patient.

Outcome Measures for Evaluating COPD Therapy

- Spirometric measure of FEV_1 to evaluate airflow limitation and inhibition of long-term lung function decline seen in COPD.
- Number (decrease in) of exacerbations and hospitalizations.
- Relief of symptoms.
- Improvement in quality of life.
- Increase in performance status.
- Increase in life expectancy.

WRITING

Directions: Answer the following question based on the reading selection. Remember to use the following writing strategies:

- Organize ideas.
- Write the first draft.
- Revise, edit, and proofread to write the final draft.

Compare the advantages and disadvantages of the two generations of antihistaminic drugs.

COMPREHENSION QUESTIONS

Directions: Answer the multiple choice questions based on the selection. Use the strategies you learned for answering multiple choice questions.

1. Iodinated glycerol is an example of
    a. Narcotic
    b. Mucolytic
    c. Vaccine
    d. Antibiotic

2. Which is contraindicated in COPD?
    a. homeopathy
    b. bronchodilators
    c. vasodilators
    d. vaccines

3. The dose of prednisolone recommended for patient's whose baseline FEV is less than 50% predicted
    a. 10 mg for 4 days
    b. 10 mg for 10 days
    c. 40 mg for 40 days
    d. 40 mg for 10 days

4. The G in GOLD guidelines stands for
    a. global
    b. good
    c. glucocorticoids
    d. gas

5. All COPD patients are recommended
    a. influenza vaccine
    b. short acting bronchodilators
    c. rehabilitation
    d. surgical treatment

6. The O in COPD stands for
    a. oral
    b. oxygen
    c. obstructive
    d. organic

7. Which is an outcome measure for COPD?
    a. monitor fluid balance
    b. relief of symptoms
    c. consider antibiotics
    d. identify and treat associated conditions

8. Which medication is central to symptom management in COPD?
   a. vaccines
   b. mucolytics
   c. antibiotics
   d. bronchodilators

9. FVC means
   a. four vector complications
   b. free viral condition
   c. forced vital capacity
   d. frequent violent coughing

10. Theophylline is an example of a:
   a. antioxidant agent
   b. bronchodilator
   c. glucocorticoid
   d. vaccine

WORD PROBLEM

Directions: Use the strategies you learned for solving word problems to answer the following question.

Steven Everfore is taking triprolidine once every four hours. If his first dose was taken at 10:00 AM, when should he take his third dose?

References

Beaver BV: *Feline behavior: a guide for veterinarians*, ed 2, St. Louis, 2003, Saunders.

Bird DL, Robinson DS: *Torres and Ehrlich modern dental assisting*, ed 8, St. Louis, 2005, Saunders.

Chabner DE: *The language of medicine*, ed 7, St. Louis, 2004, Saunders.

Diehl MO: *Diehl and Fordney's medical transcription: techniques and procedures*, ed 5, St. Louis, 2002, Saunders.

Flynn JC: *Procedures in phlebotomy*, ed 3, St. Louis, 2005, Saunders.

LaFleur Brooks M, Gillingham EA: *Health unit coordinating*, ed 5, St. Louis, 2004, Saunders.

Henry MC, Stapleton ER: *EMT prehospital care*, ed 3, St. Louis, 2004, Mosby/JEMS.

Lewis N (Ed.): *Roget's new pocket thesaurus in dictionary form*, New York, 1978, Washington Square Press.

McCurnin DM, Bassert JM: *Clinical textbook for veterinary technicians*, ed 6, St. Louis, 2006, Saunders.

Mosby's dictionary of medicine, nursing & health professions, ed 7, St. Louis, 2006, Mosby.

Purtilo RB: *Ethical dimensions in the health professions*, ed 4, Philadelphia, 2005, Saunders.

Rau JL: *Respiratory care pharmacology*, ed 6, St. Louis, 2002, Mosby.

Robinson DS, Bird DL: *Ehrlich and Torres essentials of dental assisting*, ed 3, Philadelphia, 2001, Saunders.

Solomon EP: *Introduction to human anatomy and physiology*, ed 2, St. Louis, 2003, Saunders.

Sorrentino SA: *Mosby's textbook for nursing assistants*, ed 6, St. Louis, 2004, Mosby.

Young AP, Kennedy DB: *Kinn's the medical assistant: an applied learning approach*, ed 9, St. Louis, 2003, Saunders.

Glossary

abuse harmful treatment.

academic having to do with school or learning.

accredited credentialed.

analyzing breaking down a whole into its parts.

aneurysm a sac formed by the localized dilation of the wall of an artery, vein, or the heart.

aneurysmectomy surgical removal of an aneurysm.

anxiety emotional pain.

apprenticeship the practical experience of training under skilled workers.

approximate nearly the same or nearly correct.

asepsis the absence of germs (Mosby's Dictionary, ed 7, p 150).

attending physician a doctor who works in a teaching hospital.

audience the people who will read your writing.

autocratic pertaining to one who has total power.

battered bruised.

beneficence kindness.

brainstorming spontaneously forming ideas.

cardiac pertaining to the heart (Miller-Keane, p. 250).

caret a punctuation mark that shows in what place something must be inserted.

chaotic pertaining to being in a state of utter confusion.

choppy short sentence.

chronological arranged in order of time.

common belonging to or shared by two or more mathematical entities.

comparison showing similarities of two or more items.

complement to complete or make perfect.

concentrate focus.

concepts ideas.

conclusions outcomes or results.

condensing making something more compact.

confidence self-assurance.

content the material to be learned in a course.

context the words around an unknown word that are used to figure out the meaning of the unknown word.

conventional traditional.

conversion the act of changing or transforming.

coworkers fellow employees.

credentials diplomas or certificates.

data factual information, usually in number form.

delete remove.

denominator the part of a fraction below the line that signifies division.

detect to see.

diabetes mellitus a complex disorder of carbohydrate, fat, and protein metabolism that is primarily a result of a deficiency or complete lack of insulin secretion by the beta cells of the pancreas or resistance to insulin (Mosby's Dictionary, ed 7, p 548).

diagonal passing from the upper left to the lower right or the upper right to the lower.

disclosure something made known.

discombobulated confused or upset.

distracted to have attention taken away.

document informational paper.

draft a rough version of written work.

E-mail electronic mail, a message sent on a computer.

efficiently pertaining to being productive without any waste.

emphasis stresses the importance of something.

endangered subject to being destroyed.

equation a mathematical expression of similarity.

ethicist a person who studies morality.

expanded expressed in greater detail.

exponent a mathematical number written to the right and above a number to show the raising of a power.

extends stretch forward.

external outside the body.

focused directed.

form the medium for the written message.

formulate devise.

function keys special control keys on the computer keyboard.

gastrointestinal pertaining to the stomach and intestine.

goals aims, intentions.

hemostasis stopping blood flow by natural or artificial means.

highlight emphasize.

hormone a complex chemical substance produced in one part or organ of the body that initiates or regulates the activity of an organ or group in another part (Mosby's Dictionary, ed 7, p 901).

host an animal or plant that harbors and provides sustenance for another organism.

hypertrophy increase in volume of a tissue or organ produced entirely by enlargement of existing cells.

hypotension lowered blood pressure.

identical the same.

imperative essential.

inadequate not good enough.

indentation the division of a document to create sections.

indicate demonstrate.

ingested taken in.

interfere to get in the way of.

internal inside the body.

intimidated made timid or fearful.

inverse opposite.

invoice a list showing items purchased and how much money is owed.

ions charged particles.

journal an account of daily events.

juggling dealing with several things at one time.

logically relating to the ability to use reason.

lymph a thin watery fluid originating in the organs and tissues of the body that circulates through the lymphatic vessels and is filtered by the lymph nodes (Mosby's Dictionary, ed 7, p 1123).

mechanics punctuation, sentence style, word choice, capitalization, grammar.

microcapillary tiny vessels connecting arterioles and venules.

microorganisms an organism that is too small to be seen with the unaided eye.

mobilize to put into action.

molecule the smallest unit that exhibits the properties of an element or compound.

monitoring asking yourself if you are understanding what you are reading; watching; observing.

narrating telling a story.

neurologist a physician who specializes in the nervous system and its disorders (Mosby's Dictionary, ed 7, p 1283).

numerator the part of a fraction above the line that signifies division.

objective lack of feeling toward or against.

obligation a commitment to acting in certain ways.

opponents those who disagree.

ovum egg.

pancreas a large gland located behind the stomach.

passive not active.

pathogenic having the ability to cause disease.

plaque food debris on tooth that fosters bacteria.

portable able to carry easily.

presentation the appearance.

prewriting plan for writing.

prioritize in order of importance.

procedure steps taken in a logical manner to accomplish something.

process the several steps involved in doing something.

procrastination delaying what needs to be done.

product the answer in a multiplication problem.

product the end result of the creative effort of writing.

protein any of a large group of naturally occurring complex organic nitrogenous compounds (Mosby's Dictionary, ed 7, p 1543).

pulse rate the pressure on the arteries used for the counting of heart beats.

purpose why the author is writing.

quadrants one of four parts.

quadrupled made four times greater.

quantity total amount.

quotient the answer in a division problem.

radiation energy carried by waves or a stream of particles.

recreational having to do with activities designed for relaxation and fun.

reference a book containing information, like an encyclopedia or dictionary.

resistant tending to oppose.

respectively in the given order.

reverse to go in an opposite direction.

revision rewriting.

rote use of memory mechanically.

secrete to synthesize and release a substance.

sequence the order of events.

slanted biased.

sodium salt.

statistic numerical data.

subject the topic.

subject area to be learned.

sum the answer in an addition problem.

supine lying horizontally on the back (Mosby's Dictionary, ed 7, p 1795).

syllables parts of a word that contain at least one consonant and one vowel.

tedious boring.

tendency leaning toward.

topical pertaining to the surface of a part of the body (Mosby's Dictionary, ed 7, p 1866).

transmission passage or transfer of a disease from one individual to another.

typical having the nature or being part of a type.

utility usefulness.

vague not clearly stated.

values numerical quantities.

variable a symbol representing a number that may have any value.

venipuncture the transcutaneous puncture of a vein by a sharp rigid stylet or cannula carrying a flexible plastic catheter or by a steel needle attached to a syringe or a catheter (Mosby's Dictionary, ed 7, p 1948).

veracity truthfulness.

veterinary relating to the diagnosis and cure of disease in animals.

visualize to make a mental picture.

welts a lump on the body caused by a heavy blow.

Answer Key

CHAPTER 1

Vocabulary Check

1. efficiently
2. asepsis
3. lymph
4. topical
5. neurologist
6. supine
7. autocratic
8. hemostasis
9. document
10. conclusions

Exercise 1–1

1. L
2. A
3. I
4. I
5. L
6. A
7. A
8. L
9. L
10. I

Exercise 1–2

1. protected health information
2. hemostasis
3. checking references
4. cats and psychotherapy
5. appointment scheduling

Exercise 1–3

1. Topic = The cell.
   Main idea = The cell is the basic unit of all living things.
2. Topic = Connective tissue fibers.
   Main idea = Collagen fibers are the most numerous.
3. Topic = Liquid topical anesthetics.
   Main idea = (unstated).
   Answers may vary, but they should contain the following ideas:
   Liquid topical anesthetics can be used for numbing and relieving pain in the mouth.

4. Topic = Microprocessor
   Main idea = It is the central unit of the computer that carries out the instructions of a computer's programs.
5. Topic = Preparing surgical site.
   Main idea = (unstated). Answers may vary, but they should contain the following ideas:
   Before surgery and after the animal is anesthetized, the hair should be clipped and the skin in and around the surgical site should be scrubbed with a special skin preparation.

Exercise 1–4

1. b
2. a
3. a and d
4. a
5. c

Exercise 1–5

Answers may vary, but they should include the following ideas:

- "Will you wait, or should I have the doctor call you back?"
- "I am sorry, but the doctor is still busy."
- "I am sorry that you are waiting so long. Would you like me to return your call when the doctor is free?"
- "Thank you for waiting."
- "Will you please wait while I get the information?"

Exercise 1–6

I
G
D
A
C
E
H
B
F
K
J

CHAPTER 2

Vocabulary Check

1. apprenticeship
2. beneficence
3. accredited
4. veracity
5. disclosure
6. sodium
7. quadrants
8. aneurysm
9. aneurysmectomy
10. pancreas

Exercise 2–1

See below

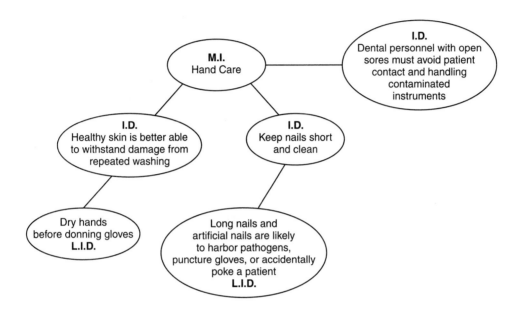

Exercise 2–2

1. b par #1
   line 2-4
2. d par #4
   line 2-3
3. c par #3
   line 8-10
4. d par #2
   line 5-9
5. a par #1
   line 3-4

Exercise 2–3

1. How to prepare a monthly billing statement.
2. 5
3. first, after, later
4. 1, 4, 5, 3, 2

Exercise 2–4

1. Sequence
2. Mixing a two-paste final impression material
3. 8
4. 3, 1, 5, 2, 4

Exercise 2–5

1. Classification
2. Yes
3. Quadrants of the abdominopelvic area or quadrants of the abdomen
4. 4
5. Right upper quadrant
   Right lower quadrant
   Left upper quadrant
   Left lower quadrant
6. Right upper quadrant

Exercise 2–6

1. Classification
2. Yes
3. Divisions of the back (spinal column)
4. 1
5. 2

Exercise 2–7

1. Examples and illustration
2. High blood pressure in arteries
3. 140/90 mm Hg

4. Diuretics, beta-blockers, ACE inhibitors, calcium channel blockers, losing weight, limiting salt intake, stopping smoking, reducing fat in diet.
5. essential, secondary

Exercise 2–8

1. Comparison-contrast
2. An argument against disclosure vs. arguments favoring disclosure
3. Honesty
   Death not taboo
   Caring entails sharing information
4. Maintain hope of patient
   Patient passive
   Benevolence
5. Answers will vary

Exercise 2–9

1. Cause-effect
2. The cause of congestive heart failure
3. Heart cannot pump required amount of blood, and blood accumulates in the lungs
4. Fluid
5. Right-sided heart failure

CHAPTER 3

Vocabulary Check

1. context
2. vague
3. analyzing
4. hormones
5. syllable
6. inadequate
7. veterinary
8. ovum
9. pathogenic
10. microorganisms

Exercise 3–2

1. (a catheter coated with a substance that does not permit the passage of x-rays)
2. also known as oil glands
3. ("tail vein")
4. (those that are used only once)
5. a portable file

Exercise 3–3

Answers will vary.

Exercise 3–4

Discrimination that is not entirely defined by law may be just as harmful as the discrimination that is defined. This type of discrimination is often referred to as subtle discrimination. Subtle discrimination is <u>not obvious</u> and is <u>seldom expressed openly.</u> It includes <u>discrimination based on a person's appearance, values, or lifestyle or on some other personal factor.</u>

Much of the discrimination that occurs in medical facilities falls into this category. Examples include <u>discrimination against overweight people, divorced people, gay people, people receiving public assistance, and people with sexually transmitted diseases.</u> Often you may not even be aware that your words or actions reflect subtle discrimination against another.

Exercises 3–5 and 3–6

See table on page 322.

Exercise 3–7

Answers will vary.

Exercise 3–8

1. metastasis
2. boldface
3. four
4. Greece
5. One
6. adjective, verb
7. anaplasia

Exercise 3–9

1. two
2. testosterone
3. heel bone
4. acquired immune deficiency syndrome
5. abdomen

Exercises 3–10

Answers will vary.

Exercise 3–11

Answers will vary.

CHAPTER 4

Vocabulary Check

1. glossary
2. pulse rate
3. reference
4. monitoring

Exercise 3–5 and 3–6

Prefix	Definition	Example	Definition of Example	Your Example
anti	against	anti-inflammatory	something that stops inflammation	answers will vary
*dys	bad, difficult	dyslexia	difficulty with the printed word	answers will vary
*exo	outside	exoskeleton	external skeleton, shell	answers will vary
*hem, hemato	relating to the blood	hemodiagnosis	blood used for diagnostic purposes	answers will vary
*hyper	over, above, beyond	hyperkinesia	above normal motor activity	answers will vary
inter	between	intersession	time between academic semesters	answers will vary
mal	poor, bad	maladjusted	poorly adjusted	answers will vary
*peri	around, near	perigastric	near the stomach	answers will vary
semi	half	semiretired	working only half-time	answers will vary
tele	distant, far	telescope	instrument for seeing objects at a distance	answers will vary

Root				
*arthro, arthr	joint	arthritis	inflammation on the joint	answers will vary
bio	life	biology	study of life forms	answers will vary
*cardi, cardio	heart	cardiopathy	disease of the heart	answers will vary
*derm, dermo	skin	dermatitis	inflammation of the skin	answers will vary
fac, fact	make, do	factory	place where objects are made	answers will vary
*path	disease	pathologist	a person who studies the disease process	answers will vary
port	carry	portable	able to be carried	answers will vary
*psych	mind	psychiatry	field of medicine concerned with mental disorders	answers will vary
spec, spect	to look at	spectator	one who looks at something	answers will vary
vers	turn	reversible	able to be turned around	answers will vary

Suffix				
able, ible	capable of	trainable	able to be trained	answers will vary
ation	act of	sanitation	act of making sanitary	answers will vary
*ectomy	excision	hysterectomy	removal of the uterus	answers will vary
ful	full of	hateful	full of hate	answers will vary
*itis	inflammation of	bursitis	inflammation of the bursa	answers will vary
ology	study	psychology	study of the mind	answers will vary
*oma	tumor	hematoma	collection of clotted blood	answers will vary
*osis	disease	nephrosis	disease of the kidneys	answers will vary
*phobia	fear	xenophobia	fear of strangers	answers will vary
scope	see	periscope	instrument for seeing around obstacles	answers will vary

*Word parts with a medical use.

5. diabetes mellitus
6. invoice
7. approximate
8. function keys
9. attending physician
10. visualize

Exercise 4–1

Answers will vary.

Exercise 4–2

Answers will vary.

Exercise 4–3

Answers will vary.

Exercise 4–4

Some of the main points that can be included in the summary are
- Not all information from a medical record should be released to a third party.
- The attending physician should be consulted if there is a question about what information is to be released.
- Summaries, abstracts, or standardized forms can be used to release information.
- Attending physicians can receive medical information on their patients without the patients' written approval.

Exercise 4–5

Answers will vary.

Exercise 4–6

C
B
A
C
B
A

Exercise 4–7

Answers will vary.

CHAPTER 5

Vocabulary Check

1. plaque
2. ingested
3. secrete
4. ions
5. hypertrophy
6. credentials

7. discombobulated
8. statistics
9. chaotic
10. protein

Exercise 5–1

1. Clinical Textbook for Veterinary Technicians
2. Dennis M. McCurnin
3. three degrees
4. Louisiana State University
5. Elsevier Saunders
6. Joanna M. Bassert, VMD
7. Sixth edition

Exercise 5–2

1. new students of phlebotomy and those collecting blood for many years
2. topics directly related to blood collection
3. professional topics
4. glossary
5. updated and expanded review questions and answers, 100-item review examination, quick reference chart; and new and updated photographs and drawings

Exercise 5–3

1. ten chapters
2. Feline Social Behavior
3. page 215
4. Feline Locomotive Behavior
5. eight major headings

Exercise 5–4

1. abdomen
2. adventitia
3. actin
4. alphabetical
5. acid

Exercise 5–5

1. 20 Common Problems, Ethics in Healthcare
2. 2002
3. fifth edition
4. Ethical Challenges in the Management of Health Information
5. alphabetical

Exercise 5–6

1. audition
2. olfaction
3. gustation
4. touch
5. vision

Exercise 5–7

1. Letters I through L
2. page 1215f
3. seven subtopics
4. yes
5. 1236f, 1236-1238, 1237f

Exercise 5–8

Answers will vary.

Exercise 5–9

1. The characteristics of x-rays that are useful to physicians in the diagnosis and treatment of disease.
2. Six.
3. Charged particles.
4. Answers will vary.
5. Answers will vary.

Exercise 5–10

1. Answers will vary.
2. Answers will vary.

Exercise 5–11

1. DNA.
2. DNA controls not only the production of new cells but also the cell's ability to grow.
3. When a cell reproduces itself.
4. DNA is located in the nucleus of a cell.
5. By directing the making of new proteins, DNA copies itself.

Exercise 5–12

1. Muscle separating the chest and abdomen
2. Breathing in
3. Breathing out
4. How the diaphragm helps the breathing process

Exercise 5–13

1. Fat-soluble Vitamins
2. Vitamin A
   Vitamin D
   Vitamin E
   Vitamin K
3. K
4. The functions, sources, and deficiency symptoms of fat-soluble vitamins
5. a. Answers will vary.
   b. Answers will vary.

Exercise 5–14

1. The Role of Nutrition in Preventive Dentistry.
2. No written answer required.

3. a. The desire to learn.
   b. The development of knowledge or skill.
4. 1/5
5. Answers will vary.
6. Answers will vary.
7. No written answer required.
8. Motivate.
9. Hard Facts About Soft Drinks.
10. It shows the reasons to limit soda consumption.
11. Answers will vary.
12. Answers will vary.
13. Answers will vary.
14. Answers will vary.

CHAPTER 6

Vocabulary Check

1. prewriting
2. process
3. form
4. purpose
5. narrating
6. E-mail
7. subject
8. audience
9. brainstorming
10. abuse

Exercise 6–1

Answers will vary.

Exercise 6–2

Answers will vary.

Exercise 6–3

Answers will vary.

Exercise 6–4

Answers will vary.

Exercise 6–5

Answers will vary.

Exercise 6–6

Answers will vary.

Exercise 6–7

Answers will vary.

Exercise 6–8

Subject **Patient with head wound**
Main Idea **Patient had sustained blood loss due to head wound.**
Purpose **Description**
Form **Case history**
Audience **Hospital emergency staff**

Subject **Patient charts**
Main Idea **To describe the purpose and format of patient charts**
Purpose **Describing**
Form **Summary**
Audience **Person learning about patient charts**

Subject **Cardiac arrest**
Main Idea **Types of cardiac arrest and treatment**
Purpose **Explanation**
Form **Descriptions**
Audience **EMTs**

CHAPTER 7

Vocabulary Check

1. product
2. draft
3. confidence
4. revision
5. expanded
6. endangered
7. slanted
8. sequence
9. detect
10. emphasis

Exercise 7–1

Answers will vary.

Exercise 7–2

Answers will vary.

Exercise 7–3

Answers will vary.

Exercise 7–4

Answers will vary.

Exercise 7–5

Answers will vary.

Exercise 7–6

Answers will vary.

Exercise 7–7

Answers will vary.

Exercise 7–8

Answers will vary.

CHAPTER 8

Vocabulary Check

1. focused
2. delete
3. mechanics
4. imperative
5. resistant
6. tedious
7. choppy
8. presentation
9. battered
10. welts

Exercise 8–1

Answers will vary.

Exercise 8–2

Both children had been battered. In the last month, two of the seven reported cases of child abuse were from middle class homes with both parents. Therefore it is imperative that you report all cases of suspected child abuse. No.
Answers will vary.

Exercise 8–3

Answers will vary.

Exercise 8–4

Answers will vary.

Exercise 8–5

1. copied
2. poked
3. neighbor
4. guardian
5. handkerchief
6. easier
7. hopeless
8. judgment
9. temperature
10. dried

Exercise 8–6

1. Who's
2. stationery
3. principal
4. chose
5. except
6. They're
7. allowed
8. too
9. dessert
10. lose

Exercise 8–7

1. fragment
2. correct sentence
3. fragment
4. run-on
5. run-on
6. correct sentence
7. fragment
8. correct sentence
9. run-on
10. fragment

Exercise 8–8

1. noun
2. preposition
3. pronoun
4. adjective
5. verb
6. interjection
7. adverb
8. interjection

Exercise 8–9

1. live
2. were
3. is
4. his
5. they
6. it
7. expects
8. her
9. his
10. follows

Exercise 8–10

Rosa is taking **E**nglish lessons so that she will be able to get a better job. She is hoping to improve her skills in reading, writing, and conversation. **W**hen she finishes this course, she will be able to enter a community college. Will this course give her skills she needs to succeed**?**

She will have to meet the following requirements**:** taking notes, understanding lectures, and comprehending her textbooks. **R**osa hopes to become a technician when she moves to **P**hiladelphia in two years**.**

CHAPTER 9

Vocabulary Check

1. values
2. typical
3. reverse
4. numerator
5. diagonal
6. denominator
7. conversion
8. common
9. caret
10. comparison

Exercise 9-1

see Table 9-1

Exercise 9–2

1. 1/4
2. 24
3. 128/14 or 64/7
4. 2/11
5. 27/28
6. 1/6
7. 2/3
8. 1/10
9. 6
10. 3 1/8

Exercise 9–3

1. 14.326
2. 8.807
3. 15.889
4. 41.35
5. 471.635
6. 0.7524404
7. 280
8. 400
9. 1/50, 4/5, 9/20
10. 0.8, 0.075, 0.2

Exercise 9–4

1. 1/2, 0.5
2. 12½%, 1/8
3. 16 ⅔%, 0.16 ⅔
4. 70%, 7/10

5. 3/5, 0.6
6. 40%, 0.4
7. 66 2/3%. 2/3
8. 37 ½%, 0.375
9. 4/5, 0.8
10. 25%, 0.25
11. 6
12. 112 ½%
13. 120
14. 37 ½%
15. 18.75

Exercise 9–5

1. 10:400 = 1:40, 1/40, 1 to 40
2. 5:20 = 1:4, 1/4, 1 to 4
3. 48:6 = 8:l, 8, 8 to l
4. 19.209 = 19/209, 19 to 209 or 1 to 11
5. 15:35 = 3:7, 3/7, 3 to 7

Exercise 9–6

1. 4:12 = 1:3 4/12 = 1/3
2. 16:40 = 2:5 16/40 = 2/5
3. 35:30 = 7:6 35/30 – 7/6
4. 108:24 = 9:2 108/24 = 9/2
5. 77:99 = 7:9 77/99 =7/9

Exercise 9–7

1. 8
2. 7
3. 81
4. 3
5. 63
6. 120
7. 210
8. 2040
9. 22
10. 124

CHAPTER 10

Vocabulary Check

1. exponent
2. extends
3. procedure
4. inverse
5. concentrate
6. equation
7. concepts
8. indicate
9. variable
10. identical

Exercise 10–1

1. +5
2. −12
3. +3
4. +35
5. −106
6. +555
7. +1
8. −32
9. +418
10. −1835

Exercise 10–2

1. −3
2. +15
3. +26
4. 0
5. −983
6. +579
7. +34,304
8. −64,108
9. 2,000,000
10. −1,000,000

Exercise 10–3

1. +8.
2. −21
3. −448
4. +8775
5. −2020
6. +88,000
7. +24
8. −100
9. +1008
10. −8,400,000

Exercise 10–4

1. +1/3
2. −1/5
3. 1/10
4. +0.12 or −1/8
5. +12
6. +2
7. −5
8. +4.5
9. −5
10. +2

Exercise 10–5

1. c = 16
2. p = 6
3. k = 16
4. m = 30
5. k = ¼
6. v = 10
7. b = 968
8. k = 448
9. n = 31
10. x = 5

Exercise 10–6

1. 10 inches
2. ½ inch
3. 4.75 inches
4. 14 inches
5. 50 inches
6. 1.5 inches
7. 78.5 square inches
8. 379.94 square inches
9. 1962.5 square inches
10. 0.03 14 square inches

Exercise 10–7

TYPE OF TRIANGLE	ANGLE A	ANGLE B	ANGLE C
equilateral	60	60	60
scalene	23	55	102
right (isosceles)	45	45	90
isosceles	35.5	109	35.5
scalene	18.2	66	95.8
isosceles	15	15	150
scalene	99.4	3.6	77
right	answers will vary but one angle must = 90°		
scalene	answers will vary		
isosceles	answers will vary		

Exercise 10–8

1. 20 inches
2. 42 inches
3. 37 feet
4. 51 miles
5. 400 kilometers

Exercise 10–9

1. 49 square inches
2. 4096 square feet
3. 20.25 square miles
4. 36,000,000 square kilometers
5. 7,840,000 square yards

Exercise 10–10

1. 26
2. 60 inches or 5 feet
3. 34 yards
4. 132 kilometers
5. 556 centimeters

Exercise 10–11

1. 40 square units
2. 4.75 square inches
3. 12.5 square feet
4. 378 square centimeters
5. 12 square miles

Exercise 10–12

1. 3.18 quarts
2. 19.08 quarts
3. 1.395 square inches
4. 1.55 square inches
5. 2.48 miles
6. 18.6 miles
7. 6.37 meters
8. 40.95 meters
9. 8.1 kilograms
10. 22.5 kilograms

CHAPTER 11

Vocabulary Check

1. quadrupled
2. quantity
3. quotient
4. data
5. intimidated
6. product
7. respectively
8. sum
9. logically
10. formulate

Exercise 11–1

Strategies: answers will vary
Solutions: 934 kilowatt hours; 1,553 hundred cubic feet

Exercise 11–2

1. 1088 feet per second
   186,324 miles per second 2 hours
2. How far does sound travel in 2 hours?
   How far does light travel in 2 hours?

In both conditions, treatment must be immediate because brain cells die in 3 to 4 minutes.

All nursing units have an emergency cart and fully equipped code arrest carts. It is important for the health unit coordinator to know the location of these carts.

Hospitals have personnel who report code arrests. They are employed in various hospital departments.

Exercise 14–7

Results and timing will vary.

Exercise 14–8

Answers will vary.

Exercise 14–9

Proofreading marks = Topic = Heading

What are proofreading marks? = Heading question
When copy is prepared for printing, it is corrected and marked, with correction symbols placed either in the margin or between the lines to indicate the changes to be made. If more than one marginal note is necessary, a slash mark (/) divides the notes. Either or both margins are used.

In proofreading your own copy, you may be more informal, using marginal notes only when there is no room on the single-spaced copy to indicate the change.

While you are a student, your instructor will proofread your work and may mark the copy and use marginal notes in a variety of ways. Therefore let us examine the proofreading marks as they are used formally and see how we may modify them for our own use. Your instructor may wish to add his or her marking symbols as well.

CHAPTER 15

Vocabulary Check

1. hypotension
2. obligation
3. utility
4. mobilize
5. radiation
6. transmission
7. ethicist
8. host
9. opponents
10. gastrointestinal

Exercise 15–1

1. b
2. c
3. c
4. c
5. d
6. a
7. c
8. c
9. b
10. c

Exercise 15–2

1. consequences
2. utilitarianism
3. Jeremy Bentham and John Stuart Mill
4. utilitarian
5. usefulness
6. consequences
7. a. to treat her in such a way that everyone else will be able to have the same treatment she received
   b. to live within my own conscience
8. Jeremy Bentham and John Stuart Mill
9. the best consequence overall
10. duties, rights, and responsibilities

Exercise 15–3

1. d
2. i
3. f
4. j
5. a
6. b
7. h
8. c
9. k
10. g

Exercise 15–4

1. T
2. F
3. T
4. F
5. F
6. T
7. F
8. T
9. T
10. F

Exercise 15–5

Part I
1. host
2. reservoir
3. carrier
4. incubation period
5. exposure

Part II
1. e
2. d
3. a
4. b
5. c

Part III
1. d
2. c
3. d
4. b
5. c

Part IV
1. F
2. F
3. T
4. F
5. F

Exercise 15–6

Answers will vary.

Exercise 15–7

Answers will vary.

READING SELECTION I

Preview Question

Answers will vary.

Vocabulary

Answers will vary.

Writing

Answers will vary.

Comprehension Questions
1. c
2. d
3. d
4. d
5. a
6. a
7. c
8. b
9. c
10. d

Word problem

$2916.67
$26,000
$2166.67

READING SELECTION 2

Preview Question

Answers will vary.

Vocabulary

Answers will vary.

Writing

Answers will vary.

Comprehension Questions
1. T
2. T
3. T
4. T
5. F
6. F
7. F
8. F
9. F
10. T

Word Problem

270 cassettes
30 cassettes

READING SELECTION 3

Preview Question

Epidermis: constantly renewing itself; waterproofing
Dermis: provides strength and elasticity
Superficial fascia: attaches skin to underlying tissue

Vocabulary

Answers will vary.

Writing

Answers will vary.

Comprehension Questions
1. C
2. C
3. B
4. A
5. B
6. C
7. C
8. B
9. A
10. B

Word Problem

41,200 people

READING SELECTION 4

Preview Question

Skeletal, muscular, nervous, sensory, endocrine, cardiovascular, and lymphatic systems
Answers will vary.

Vocabulary

Answers will vary.

Writing

Answers will vary.

Comprehension Questions

1. cardiac
2. 700 muscles
3. central nervous system
4. autonomic nervous system
5. axial, appendicular
6. neurotransmitters
7. cardiovascular system
8. hormones
9. waste products and carbon dioxide
10. skeletal muscle

Word Problem

approximately 3 replacements

READING SELECTION 5

Preview Question

Answers will vary.

Vocabulary

Answers will vary.

Writing

Answers will vary.

Comprehension Questions

1. c
2. a
3. b
4. d
5. a
6. c
7. b
8. c
9. d
10. d

Word Problem

5,600,000 stray cats

READING SELECTION 6

Preview Question

dentist, clinical dental assistant, expanded-functions dental assistant, dental hygienist, business assistant dental laboratory technician

Vocabulary

Answers will vary.

Writing

Answers will vary.

Comprehension Questions

1. T
2. T
3. F
4. T
5. F
6. F
7. T
8. F
9. T
10. T

Word Problem

Profit; $10,727

READING SELECTION 7

Preview Question

nose, pharynx, larynx, trachea, bronchi, lungs

Vocabulary

Answers will vary.

Writing

Answers will vary.
Comprehension Questions

1. C
2. E
3. F
4. A
5. D
6. E
7. F
8. B
9. A
10. C

Word Problem

1.7%

READING SELECTION 8

Preview Question

Drapes are folded in accordion fashion so that they are easily unfolded onto the patient.

Vocabulary

Answers will vary.

Writing

Answers will vary.

Comprehension Questions

1. neck
2. with autoclave tape
3. 10 steps
4. so they are easily unfolded onto the patient
5. 15 cm in width
6. 9 steps
7. The gown, along with a hand towel and sterilization indicator, is placed diagonally onto the nonfenestrated drapes.
8. The corners are folded over the gown.
9. 6 steps
10. contents, date, initials of the individual preparing the pack

Word Problem

8 accordion folds

READING SELECTION 9

Preview Question

1. pneumonia
2. asthma
3. emphysema

Vocabulary

Answers will vary.

Writing

Answers will vary.

Comprehension

1. T
2. F
3. T
4. T
5. T
6. T
7. F
8. T
9. F
10. T

Word Problem

1 ½ hours

READING SELECTION 10

Preview Question

A pathogen is a microorganism that is capable of causing disease.

Vocabulary

Answers will vary.

Writing

Answers will vary.

Comprehension

A. 7
B. 10
C. 8
D. 1
E. 6
F. 9
G. 5
H. 2
I. 4
J. 3

Word Problem

3,840

READING SELECTION 11

Preview Question

An intercom is a device used to communicate between the nurses' station and patients' rooms on a nursing unit.

Vocabulary

Answers will vary.

Writing

Answers will vary.

Comprehension

1. redial
2. confidential
3. pneumatic
4. fax machine
5. unit intercom
6. voice mail
7. specialty
8. twice
9. voice paging system
10. shredded

Word Problem

2 hours

READING SELECTION 12

Preview Question

General anesthesia, local anesthesia, and spinal anesthesia

Vocabulary

Answers will vary.

Writing

Answers will vary.

Comprehension

1. b
2. c
3. a
4. b
5. a
6. c
7. d
8. a
9. c
10. c

Word Problem

1:50 PM

READING SELECTION 13

Preview Question

respiratory and cardiac arrest

Vocabulary

Answers will vary.

Writing

Answers will vary.

Comprehension

1. T
2. F
3. T
4. T
5. F
6. T
7. T
8. T
9. T
10. F

Word Problem

two times the risk

READING SELECTION 14

Preview Question

Lou Gehrig's disease

Vocabulary

Answers will vary.

Writing

Answers will vary.

Comprehension

1. deterioration
2. baseball player
3. epilepsy
4. one side of the face
5. postictal
6. four
7. thymectomy
8. degeneration
9. paralysis
10. palliative

Word Problem

10 students

READING SELECTION 15

Preview Question

Chronic obstructive pulmonary disease.

Vocabulary

Answers will vary.

Writing

Answers will vary.

Comprehension

1. b
2. c
3. d
4. a
5. a
6. c
7. b
8. d
9. c
10. b

Word Problem

6:00 PM

Index

An *f* following page numbers refers to figures and a *t* refers to tables.